The Making of a Physician

The Making of a Physician

TCU's Anne Burnett Marion School of Medicine

BY LISA MARTIN

PHOTOGRAPHY BY JOYCE MARSHALL

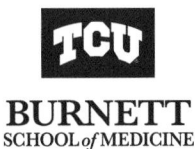

BURNETT
SCHOOL *of* MEDICINE

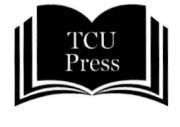

FORT WORTH, TEXAS

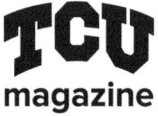

magazine

A JOINT PROJECT OF TCU MAGAZINE AND TCU PRESS

Contents

KNOWLEDGE IS POWER - SIR FRANC

아는 것이 힘이다

Tri thức là sức mạnh

SAVOIR, C'EST PO

知识就是力量

CONOCIMIENTO ES PODE

Foreword
FROM THE CHANCELLOR

At TCU, we strive for new heights by building upon the extraordinary ambition of the leaders who came before us. So many people have transformed our University with their vision, passion and generosity. The Anne Burnett Marion School of Medicine shows us, once again, what we can accomplish by working together.

The journey began when TCU Trustee Dee J. Kelly Jr. asked whether I'd considered launching a medical school. I thought about the successes of our prehealth professions and nursing programs and the incredible opportunities for medical innovation in the thriving Fort Worth community. I felt confident that our extended network of supporters would help us bring this vision for a medical school to life.

In 2016, we hired Dr. Stuart D. Flynn as founding dean of TCU's School of Medicine — the first new allopathic medical school to serve Fort Worth in more than 100 years. Dean Flynn and his imaginative team spent the next several years designing a new way of educating doctors that focused on creating Empathetic Scholars®. As our world becomes smarter, we must also seek ways to connect in meaningful ways. The curriculum at the Anne Burnett Marion School of Medicine leans into the compassion and empathy so necessary for effective medical care.

We welcomed the first class of medical students in July 2019. These future physicians arrived in Fort Worth from all over the country, with backgrounds as diverse as the specialties they would ultimately pursue. Fort Worth entrepreneur and philanthropist H. Paul Dorman covered the first year of tuition for each of the 60 students in the inaugural class, a gift that helped us recruit these high-caliber scholars to TCU.

Unflagging mentorship and innovative methods of learning, which included clinical training almost from Day 1, enabled the medical school and the Dorman Scholars — as members of the Class of 2023 will be forever known — to pivot rapidly when Covid-19 disrupted the world in early 2020.

A fully technological learning environment empowered the first-year students to become participants in real-time solutions throughout the unprecedented public health emergency. A hallmark of TCU is that we nurture leaders at all levels. The future physicians immediately made an impact on the community through a virtual blood drive and the collection and donation of personal protective equipment. In winter 2021, the students administered hundreds of vaccines to members of the community.

In March 2023, 100 percent of the first class matched to a residency program in the U.S. That's a coup for any medical school, let alone a new one. The students became doctors upon graduating eight weeks later. The following month, the Burnett School of Medicine became fully accredited (another feat), affirming that we provide the highest standards of training in health care innovation.

Our medical school will continue to positively impact North Texas with its new, more than 95,000-square-foot campus in the heart of the city's medical district. These facilities, which will foster innovation and enhance our impactful curriculum, are an exciting development in the history of the University. We've just begun to benefit from TCU's strategic campus expansion, which enhances the success of our students while at the same time improving our community's health.

Through the Anne Burnett Marion School of Medicine, TCU will be leading the way to longer, healthier lives for generations to come.

Thank you for your support and for being a part of this vision to transform health care.

— Victor J. Boschini, Jr.
10th Chancellor

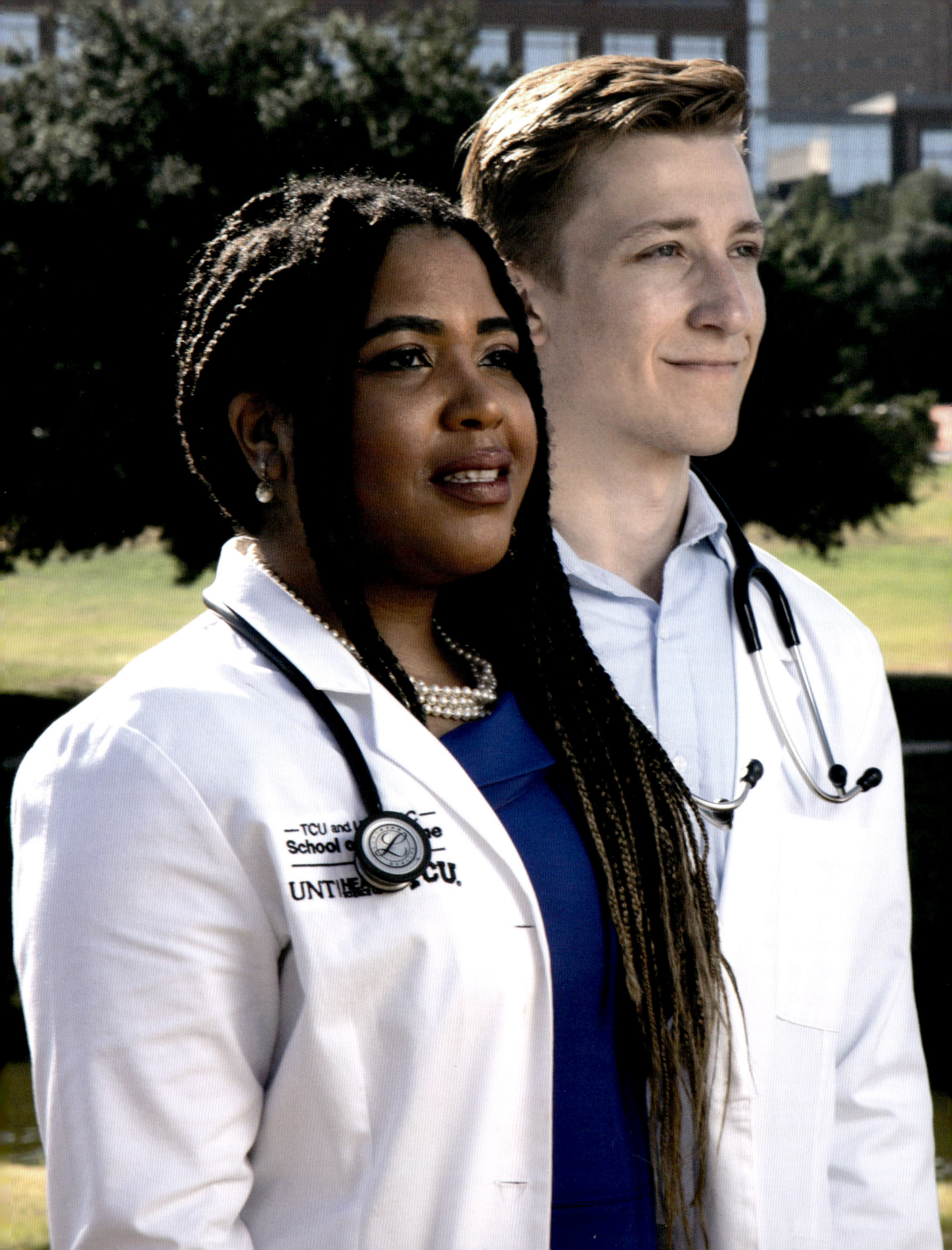

Introduction

When TCU opened the first new allopathic medical school in Fort Worth in more than 100 years, the university created a 21st-century institution that harnesses cutting-edge technology while emphasizing empathy. By centering its curriculum on patient care, the Anne Burnett Marion School of Medicine has upended longstanding models by teaching physicians-in-training to walk in their patients' shoes.

"There were missing pieces from how we have traditionally educated doctors," said Dr. Stuart D. Flynn, the medical school's founding dean. "What I would hear patients say is what they really wanted their doctor to do was sit down, look them in the eye and listen."

Flynn and his team designed a curriculum called the Compassionate Practice® to cultivate the medical students' soft skills. Strong interpersonal communication can enhance patient interactions while also elevating the physician's own experience, an area of growing concern. A national study published in July 2023 revealed that nearly a third of doctors working in hospitals felt burned out, with 23 percent wishing they could quit their jobs. The American Medical Association described burnout as a "health crisis for doctors — and patients."

"After about a week of sitting around a table in those early days, when all we were doing was talking about the kind of school we wanted to have, we realized what we wanted was to create Empathetic Scholars®," said Judy Bernas, senior associate dean and chief communication and strategy officer for the school, who coined and trademarked the term.

"People may think medical school is about the physician, but it's not," Flynn noted. "Patients are the central focus at the Burnett School of Medicine, where everything revolves around them."

"The No. 1 priority for us in the recruitment and selection of our medical students is goodness of fit for our mission and vision," said psychologist Erin Nelson, the assistant dean of physician communication at the Burnett School of Medicine. "We've worked really hard to find students whose hearts align with the spirit of our medical school, those who are drawn toward empathy and to being involved in service to others."

To advance and embolden creative thought, the school incorporates writing, active-listening training and personal reflection throughout the four-year curriculum.

"Blending a medical education with liberal arts helps shape tomorrow's physicians as ethical leaders who are skilled in interpersonal communication and nimble thinkers who thrive as part of a team to treat patients in ways that consider the whole human condition," said TCU Chancellor Victor J. Boschini, Jr.

The medical school received preliminary accreditation in fall 2018. The following July, the fastest-growing large city in the U.S. welcomed its first class of 60 students seeking their MD degrees.

Sixty percent of students in the Class of 2023

Charna Kinard, Jonas Kruse and their classmates took a chance on a new medical school with an innovative curriculum and no established reputation.

CLASS OF 2023
BY THE NUMBERS

Total students: 60

60% women
40% men

20% earned undergraduate
degrees from TCU

52% from Texas

16% arrived with
graduate-level
degrees

Average age: 24

Average college GPA:
3.62 out of 4.0

Average MCAT score:
508 out of 528

were women, with over half hailing from Texas. Sixteen percent had already earned graduate-level degrees, while a dozen students — a full 20 percent — were TCU alumni.

"We have the privilege and responsibility of educating medical leaders of the future," said Mark Johnson, chair of the TCU Board of Trustees from 2017 to 2023. "This is an extraordinary way for us to live up to our mission of responsible global citizenship, starting right here in Fort Worth."

From the outset, homegrown support proved essential to the ambitious endeavor. In 2017, Fort Worth pharmaceutical entrepreneur and philanthropist H. Paul Dorman committed to donating the first year of tuition for every member of the inaugural class.

While the Dorman Scholars, as the students collectively became known, were learning the science and art of medicine, school leaders worked with area hospitals to create opportunities for graduate-level medical education. Upon graduating from medical school after four years, every practicing physician in the U.S. must complete a residency in a specialty. The number of applicants nationwide consistently outpaces available residency slots.

In 2020, the Burnett School of Medicine partnered with Baylor Scott & White All Saints Medical Center – Fort Worth for a resident program that would grow to more than 150 physicians each year. The school also expanded its affiliation with Texas Health Resources for residency programs at hospitals in Fort Worth, Hurst-Euless-Bedford and Denton, with the goal of training more than 100 physicians annually.

The Burnett School of Medicine began building a medical campus in Fort Worth's Near Southside neighborhood in 2022. Other health care facilities in the medical district include Texas Health Harris Methodist Hospital Southwest Fort Worth, Cook Children's Medical Center and the Moncrief Cancer Institute.

"This is one of the very few projects that I have ever done where everyone was for it," Boschini said.

The more than 95,000-square-foot medical education building sits on 5 acres at the corner of South Henderson and West Rosedale streets, 3 miles north of the main campus. The state-of-the-art structure reflects the TCU look with its iconic red roofs, tan brick and distinctive exterior arches.

"The School of Medicine campus underscores our commitment to educating medical doctors and clinicians of the future to serve our large and growing community," Johnson said. "Providing an excellent academic environment and state-of-the-art facilities exemplifies the TCU experience."

"TCU is an institution of innovation," TCU President Daniel W.

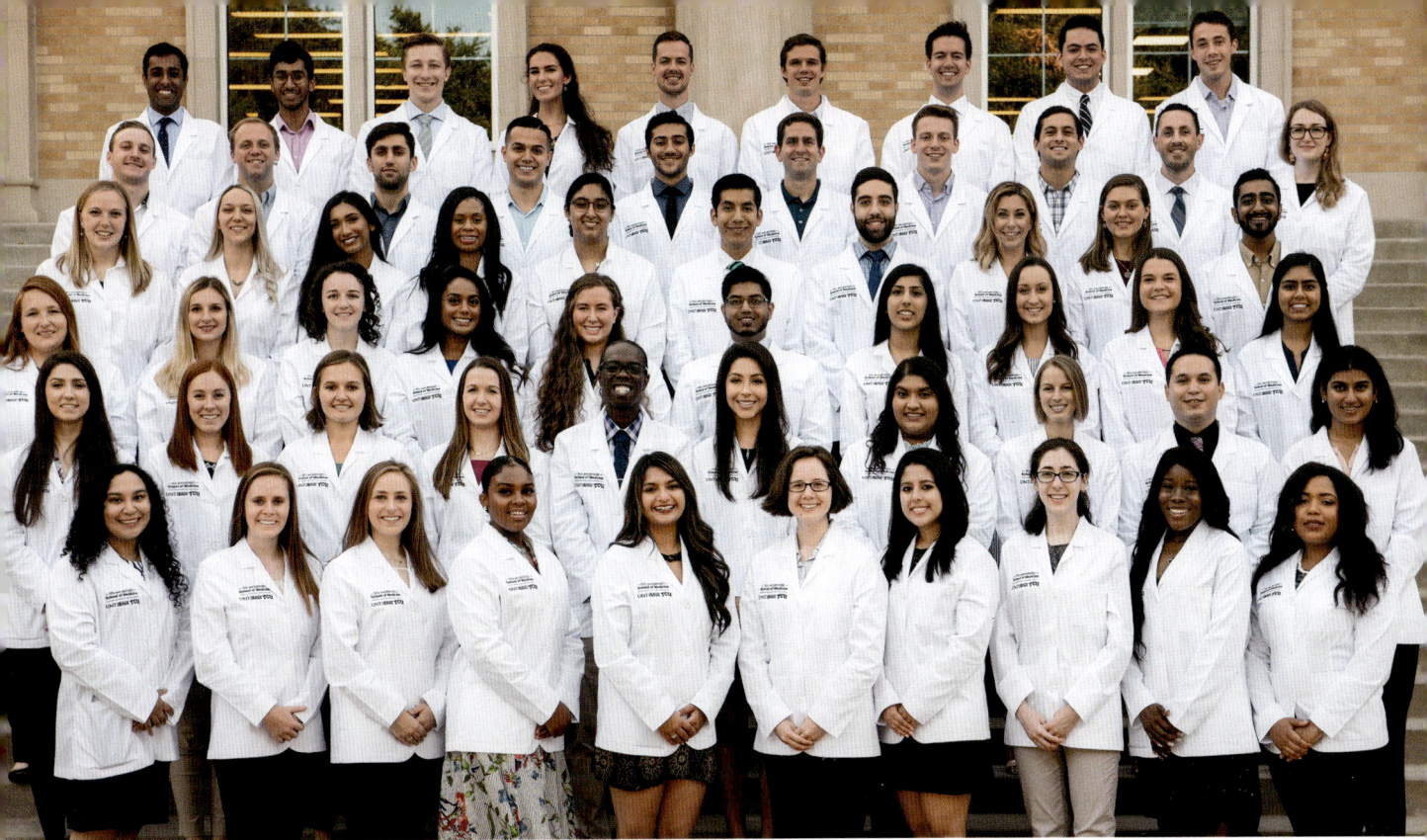

Of the 60 students in the inaugural class of the Anne Burnett Marion School of Medicine, 12 earned undergraduate degrees from TCU. In Year 1, TCU partnered with the University of North Texas Health Science Center to launch the school. TCU assumed sole ownership in January 2022.

Pullin said in spring 2023. "The new building changes the face of TCU by squarely positioning ourselves in this part of the community. It will allow us to connect and collaborate."

Flynn noted that the floor housing anatomy, simulation and clinical skills "is 100 percent patient-centered, with everything high tech and forward-looking."

Forward-thinking epitomized the school's namesake. Anne Burnett Marion (1938-2020) presided over Burnett Ranches and the Burnett Oil Co. on the historic 6666 Ranch northwest of Fort Worth. The former TCU Trustee donated a total of $50 million to the medical school, one of the few ever named for a woman.

At least half of the first four classes matriculating at the medical school were composed of women, part of a nationwide trend. In 2019, for the first time in history, the majority of medical students in the U.S. were women.

"We are training physicians who are able to explain evidence-based research to their patients and know if the science is solid," Flynn said of the school's mission. "They must know what new and innovative personal health technologies are out there and how they can be used to reach beneficial outcomes for their patients. That's the challenge and the beauty of training the next generation of physicians."

During its first year of medical school, the Class of 2023 leaned into empathy and compassion training as the Covid-19 pandemic disrupted nearly all of the new school's plans. Four years of study at TCU's medical school included rigorous courses in a range of disciplines, as well as extensive clinical experience and make-or-break standardized tests. Along the way, the students selected specialty areas for their medical careers.

To the delight of everyone associated with the school, 100 percent of TCU's fourth-year students matched to residency programs in March 2023. After

Research from the Association of American Medical Colleges indicates the U.S. could need

124,000 MORE DOCTORS

than it will have by 2034.

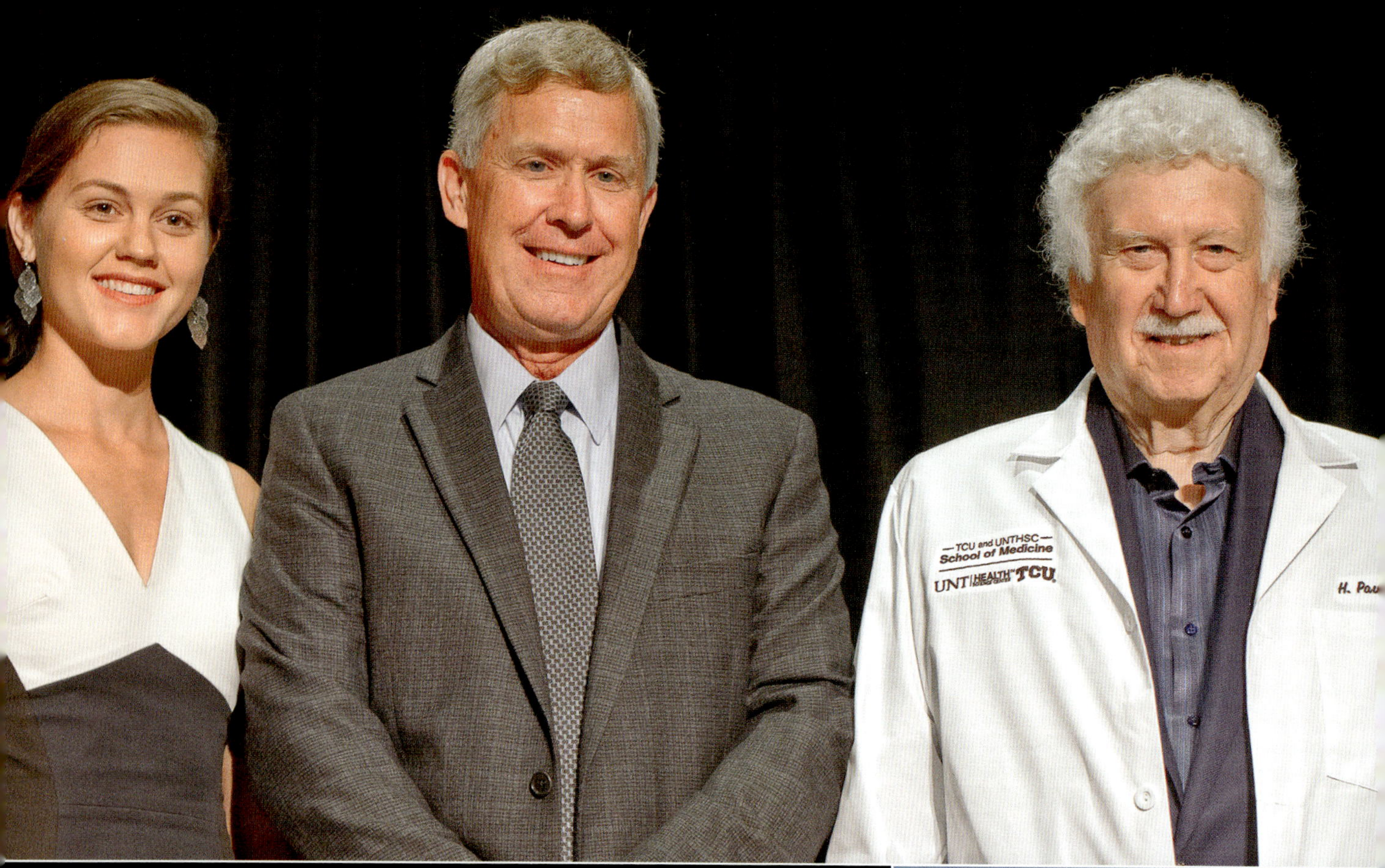

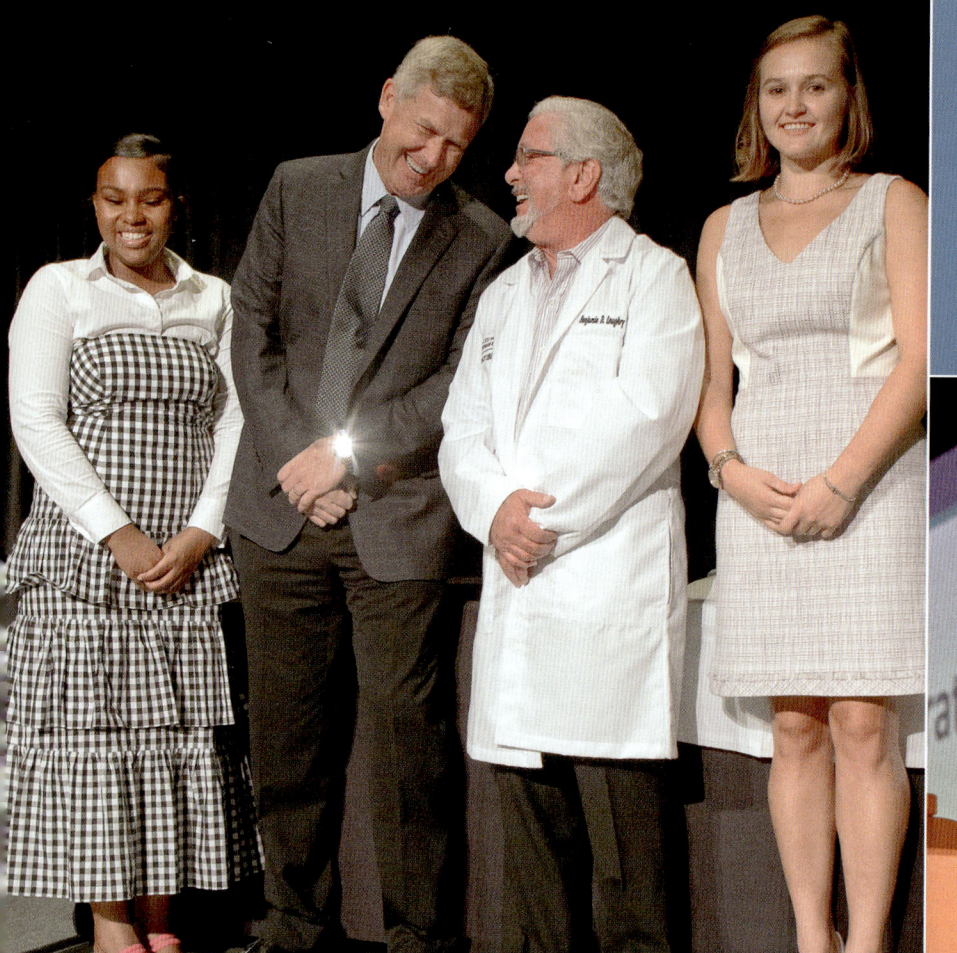

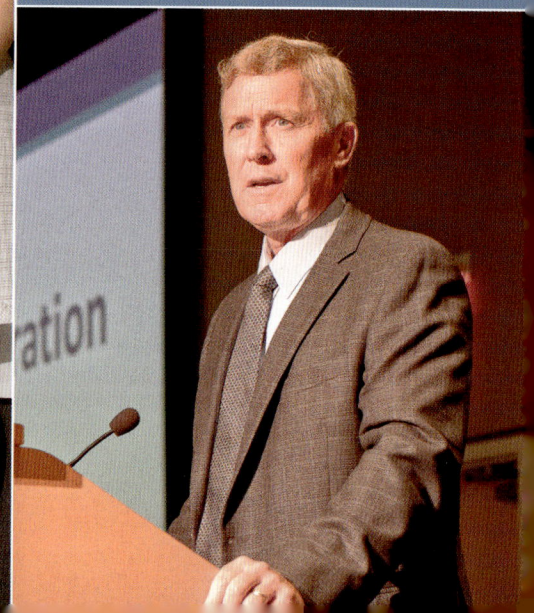

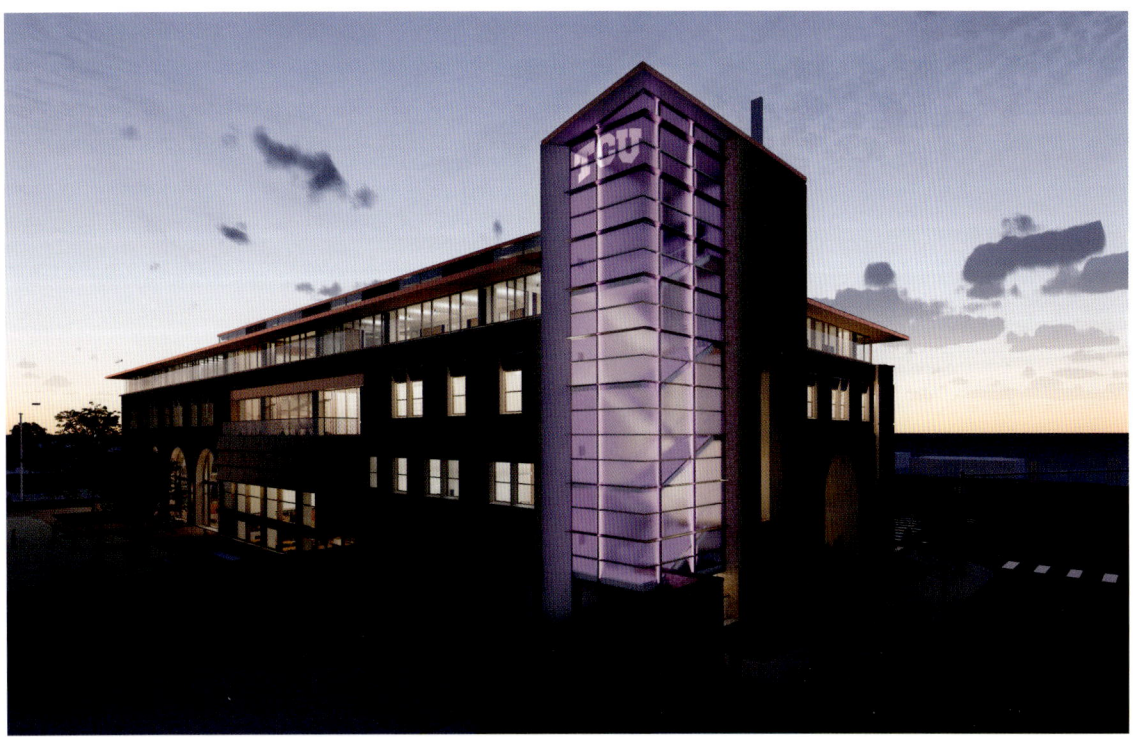

Arnold Hall, home to the Anne Burnett Marion School of Medicine at Texas Christian University, opened in summer 2024 in Fort Worth's medical district.

graduating two months later, the class scattered to universities and hospitals around the country.

The Burnett School of Medicine received full accreditation in June 2023, at the midway point of TCU's sesquicentennial celebrations. The certification was another significant milestone for the school, Boschini said. "This achievement represents the culmination of a vision that started in 2015 with a bold idea and a tremendous amount of passion."

TCU Magazine followed six students in the Class of 2023 through all four years of their medical school experience. During their time as TCU medical students, Ivette "Ive" Mota Avila, Edmundo Esparza, Charna Kinard, Jonas Kruse, Quinn Losefsky and Dilan Sunil Shah gave us unrivaled insight into their lives. They opened up to share their fears and frustrations, their struggles and triumphs, and their goals and exciting achievements.

All six formed indelible relationships with faculty, patients and classmates while forging singular paths. Each also matched to a U.S. residency in his or her top field of choice. Avila became an OB-GYN. Esparza pursued internal medicine, while Shah dedicated himself to psychiatry. Kruse chose interventional radiology, an emerging field of medicine steeped in high-tech imagining. Losefsky and Kinard fulfilled long-held ambitions of becoming surgeons.

What follows is a year-by-year look at their journey through the Anne Burnett Marion School of Medicine at TCU. ✦

Opposite page, clockwise from top: At the white coat celebration in July 2019, Quinn Losefsky and founding dean Stuart D. Flynn, center, paid tribute to Fort Worth philanthropist H. Paul Dorman, who donated the first year of tuition for the entire inaugural class; Flynn addressed students and their families at the ceremony; Ben Loughry, center right, who gifted white coats to all 60 students, shared a laugh with Flynn while Shanice Cox, left, and Shelby Wildish looked on.

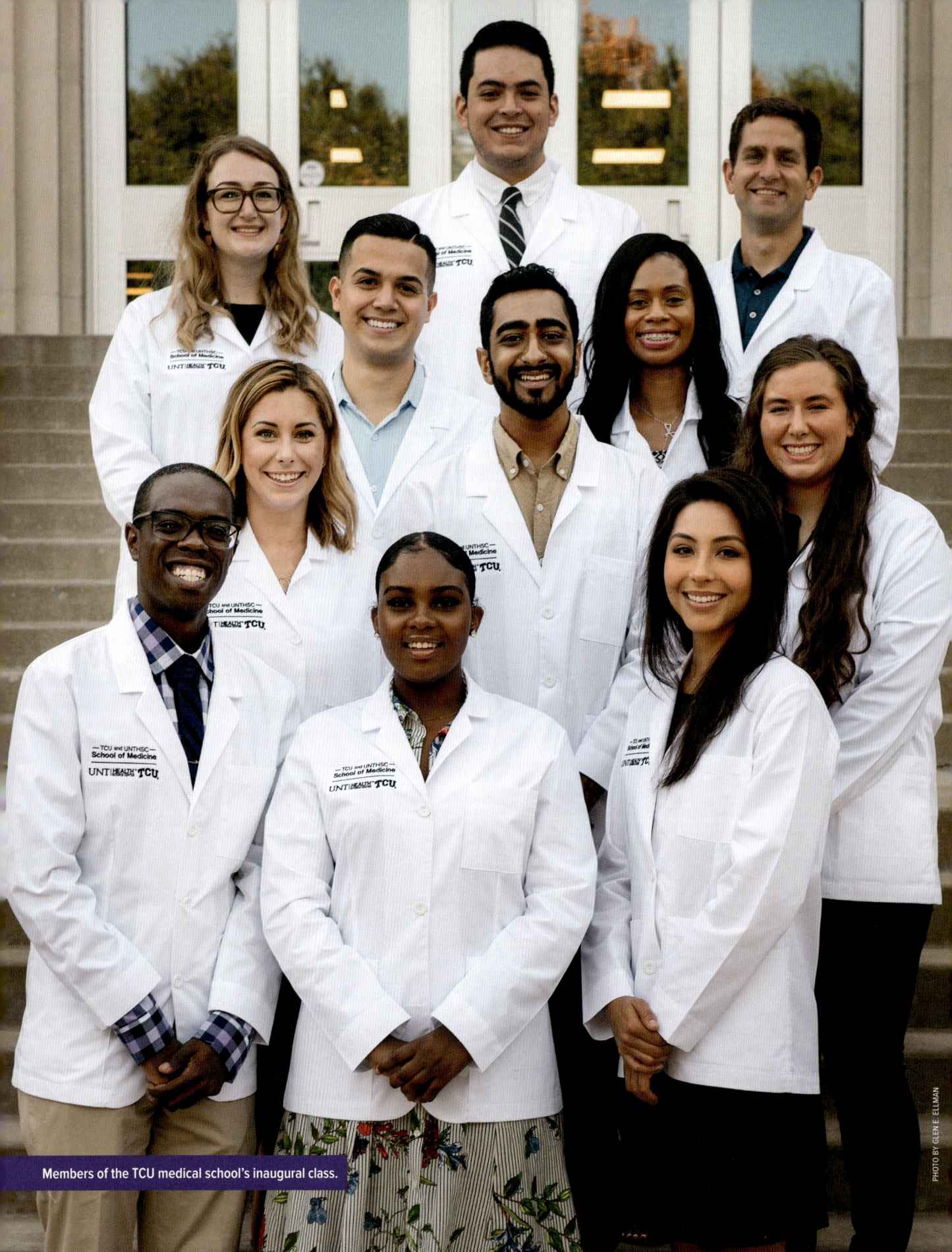

Members of the TCU medical school's inaugural class.

PHOTO BY GLEN E. ELLMAN

The Six

TCU Magazine followed six students in the Class of 2023 through their four years of medical education at the Burnett School of Medicine.

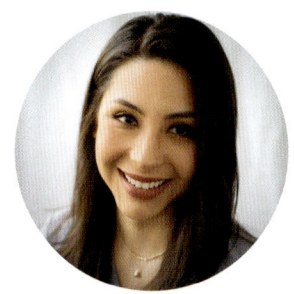

IVE MOTA AVILA

Hometown: Austin, Texas
Alma Maters: Loyola University Chicago, Southern New Hampshire University (MBA)
Specialty: Obstetrics/Gynecology

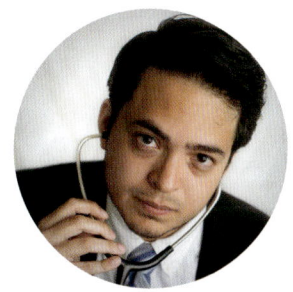

EDMUNDO ESPARZA

Hometown: El Paso, Texas
Alma Mater: The University of Texas at El Paso (BS + MBA)
Specialty: Internal Medicine

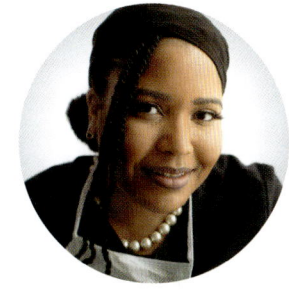

CHARNA KINARD

Hometown: Chicago, Illinois
Alma Mater: Loyola University Chicago
Specialty: General Surgery

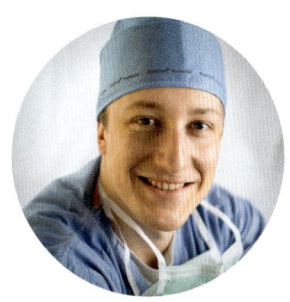

JONAS KRUSE

Hometown: San Clemente, California
Alma Mater: Baylor University
Specialty: Interventional Radiology

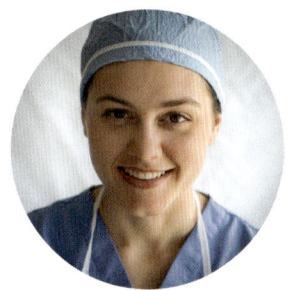

QUINN LOSEFSKY

Hometown: Austin, Texas
Alma Mater: TCU
Specialty: General Surgery

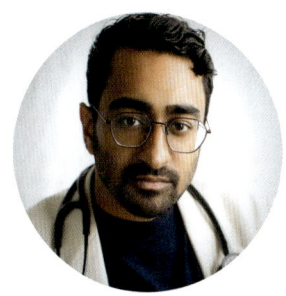

DILAN SUNIL SHAH

Hometown: McKinney, Texas
Alma Mater: Austin College
Specialty: Psychiatry

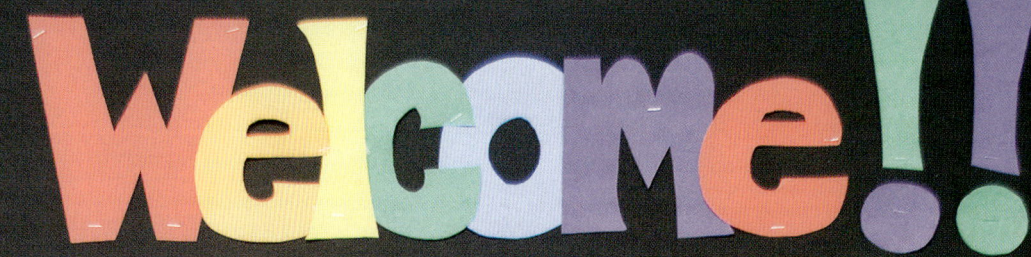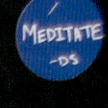

Welcome!!

CLASS OF 2023

HOW DO YOU

"DO"

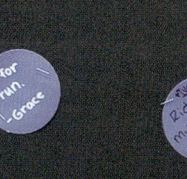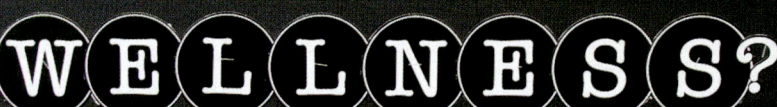

WELLNESS?

1. PICK ANY CIRCLE.
2. WRITE YOUR ANSWER.
3. STAPLE ABOVE.
4. MIX & MINGLE!

MEDITATE
My dog
podcasts
-Morgan
Working
Out
-Madison
Go for
a run.
-Grace
Ride
my horses
-baby
Punching
my stamp
Meditation!
prayer
Drawing
Dance/Yoga
-Mallory
SQUASH
Shelby
Jogging
-Helena
Cook

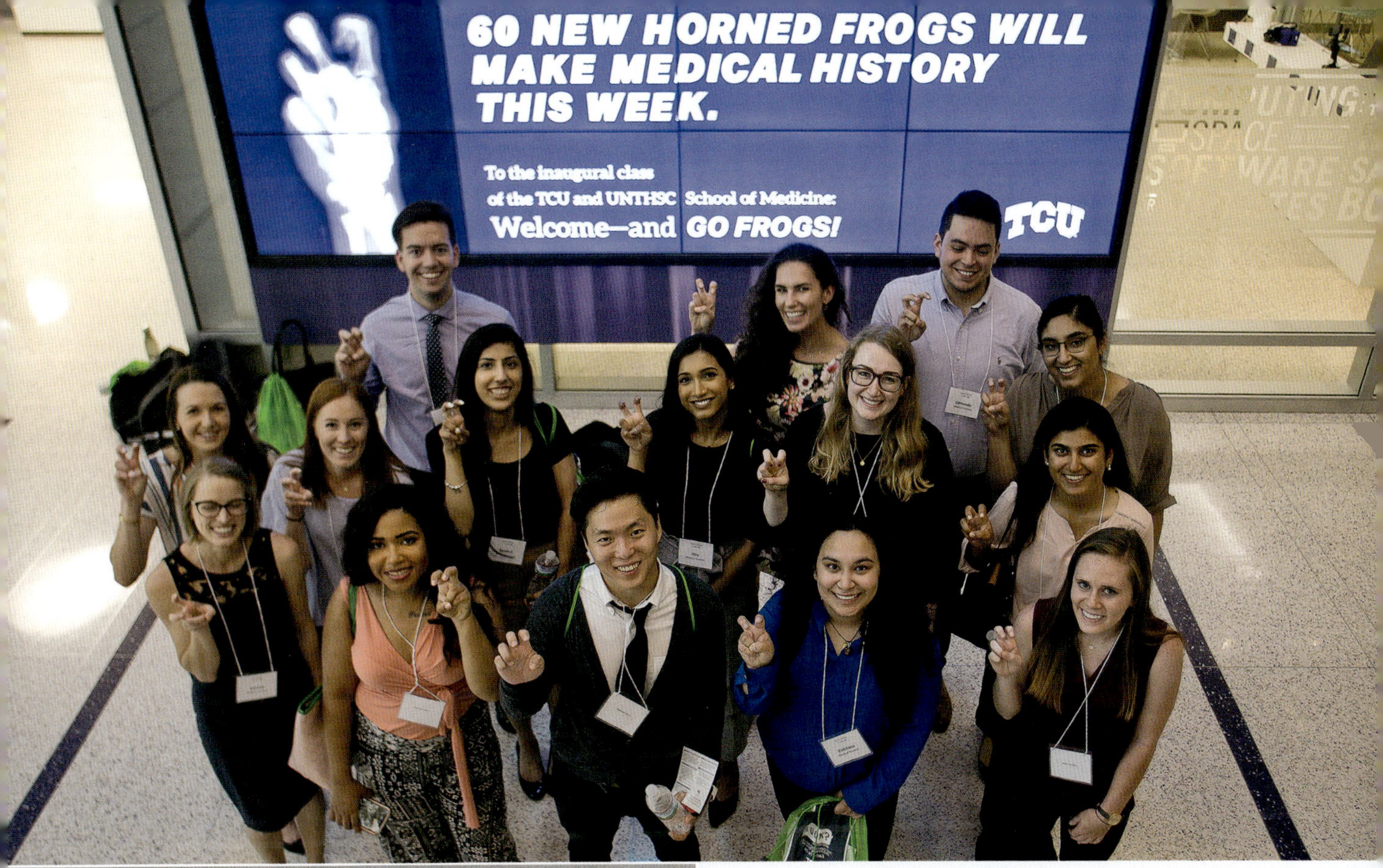

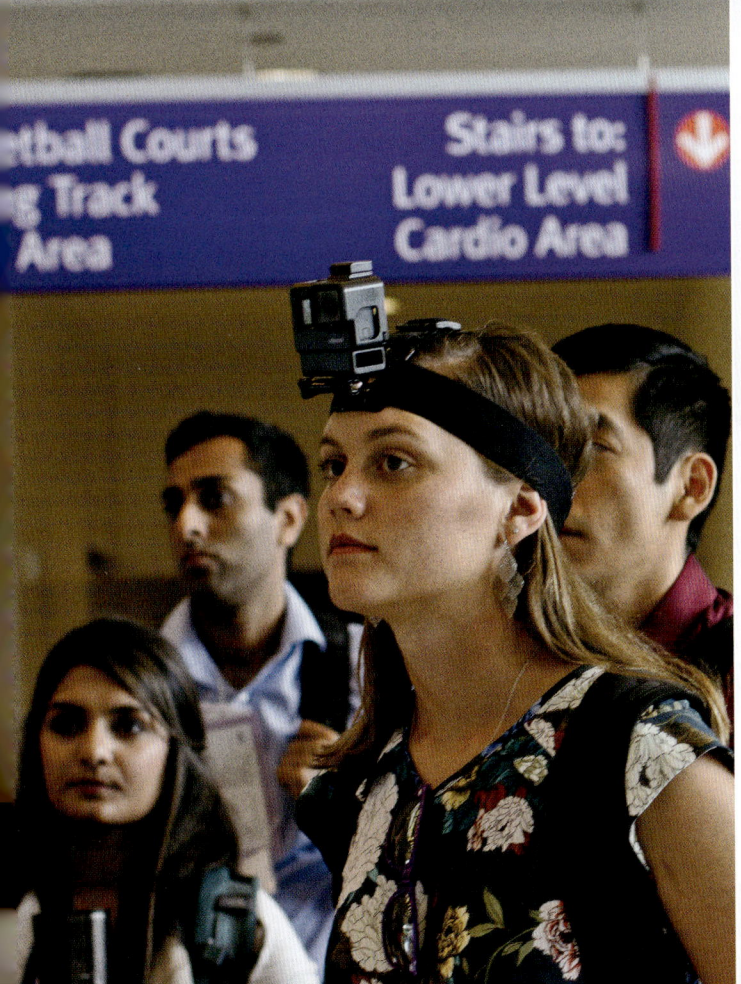

60 NEW HORNED FROGS WILL MAKE MEDICAL HISTORY THIS WEEK.

To the inaugural class
of the TCU and UNTHSC School of Medicine:
Welcome—and *GO FROGS!*

TCU

Stairs to:
Lower Level
Cardio Area

...tball Courts
...g Track
...Area

Opposite page: From Day 1 at TCU's School of Medicine, the students began to consider how they fit into a larger context of health care.

Above: Sixty students came together from around the country to form the first class of TCU's medical school. In deciding to become part of the Class of 2023, these future doctors wrote themselves into the story that began with a multiyear effort to open the first new allopathic medical school in Fort Worth in more than 100 years. During their first week of medical school in 2019, activities included a pep rally and conversations about empathy and diversity, plus practical matters like receiving their lockers.

Left: TCU grad Quinn Losefsky donned a portable camera while helping show her medical school classmates around campus.

PHOTOS BY MARK GRAHAM

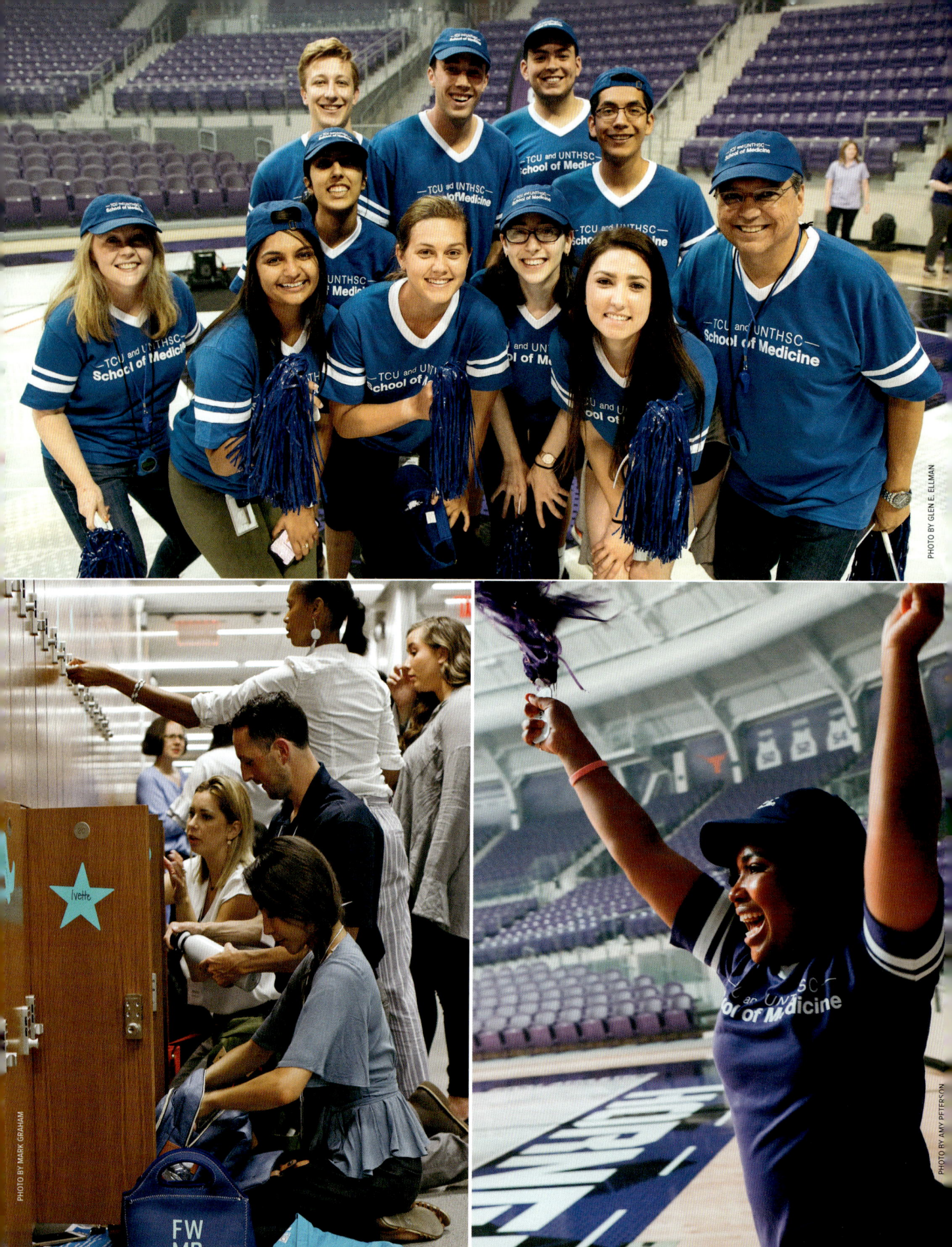

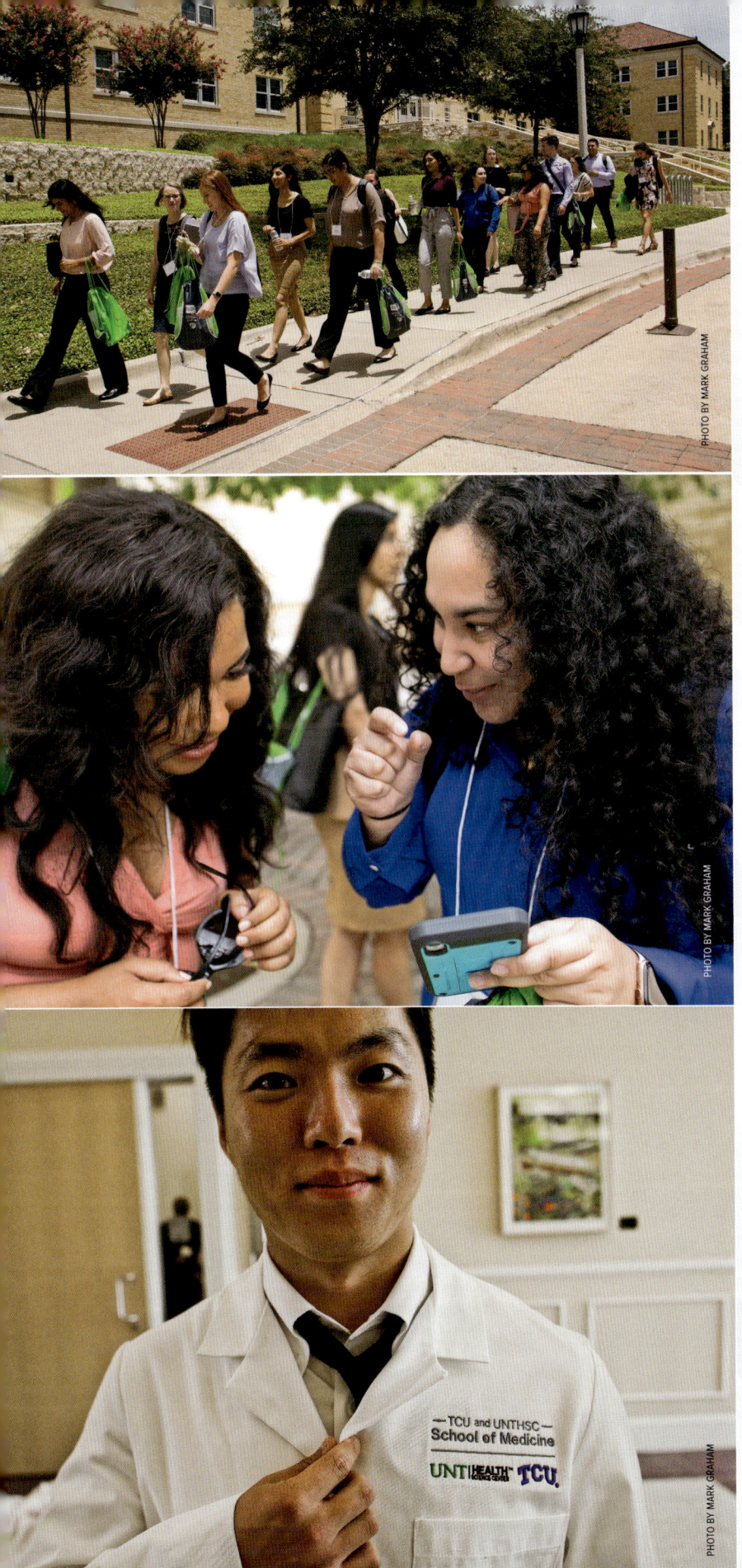

PHOTO BY MARK GRAHAM

PHOTO BY MARK GRAHAM

PHOTO BY MARK GRAHAM

Opposite page, clockwise from top:

Students were divided into 10-member teams, each overseen by two physician development coaches who worked with them all four years. The blue team met its mentors during the coaching reveal before the first semester commenced.

Charna Kinard, a fresh arrival from Chicago, was a member of the purple team.

Ive Avila, an undergraduate classmate of Kinard's, moved her belongings into her assigned medical school locker.

This page, from top:

A tour of the TCU campus was on the activity list for the first official day at the Burnett School of Medicine.

Kinard, left, and classmate Vandana Garg shared the excitement of officially being medical students.

Lucas Yoon and his fellow students sported fresh white coats in their school photo IDs.

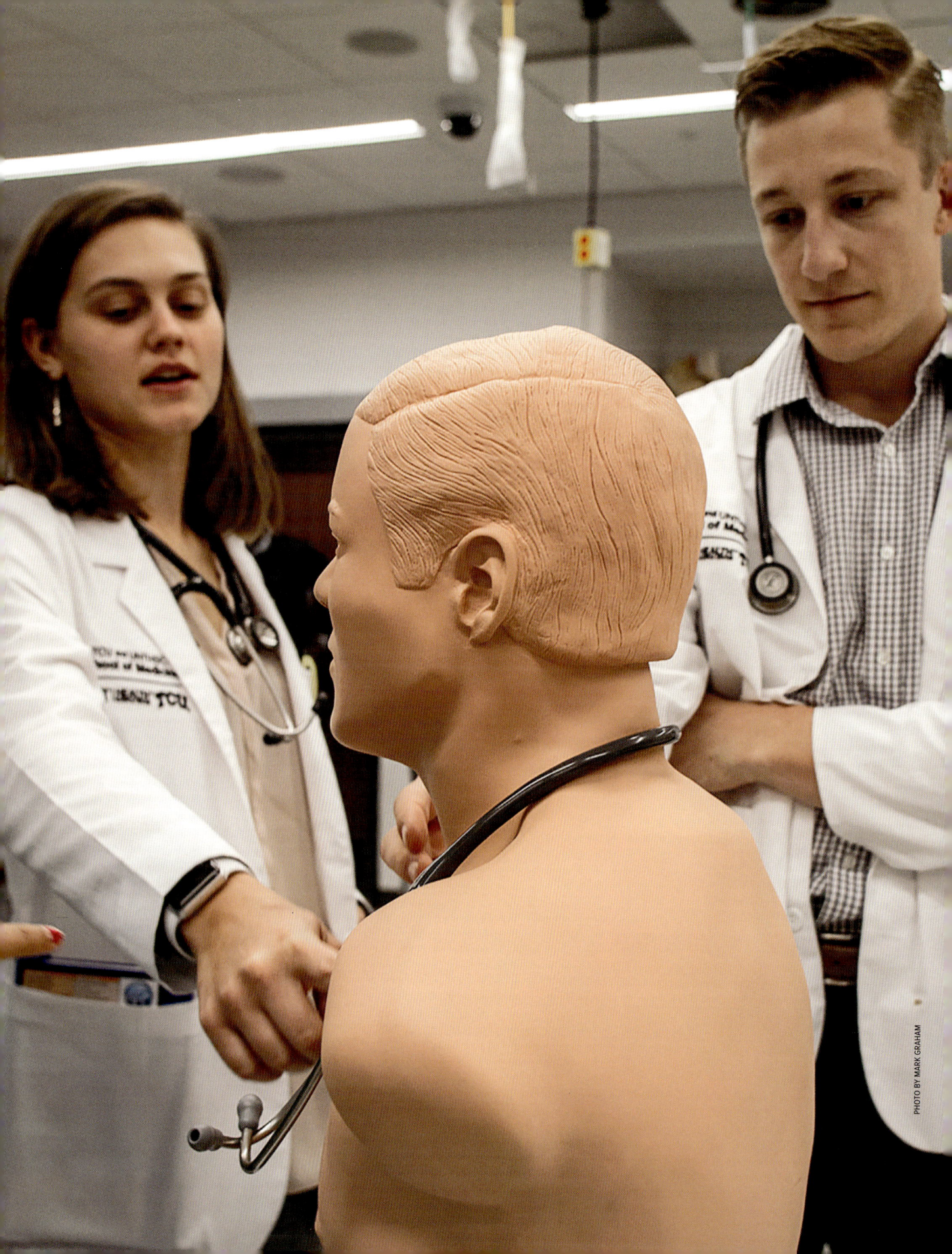

YEAR ONE

2019-20

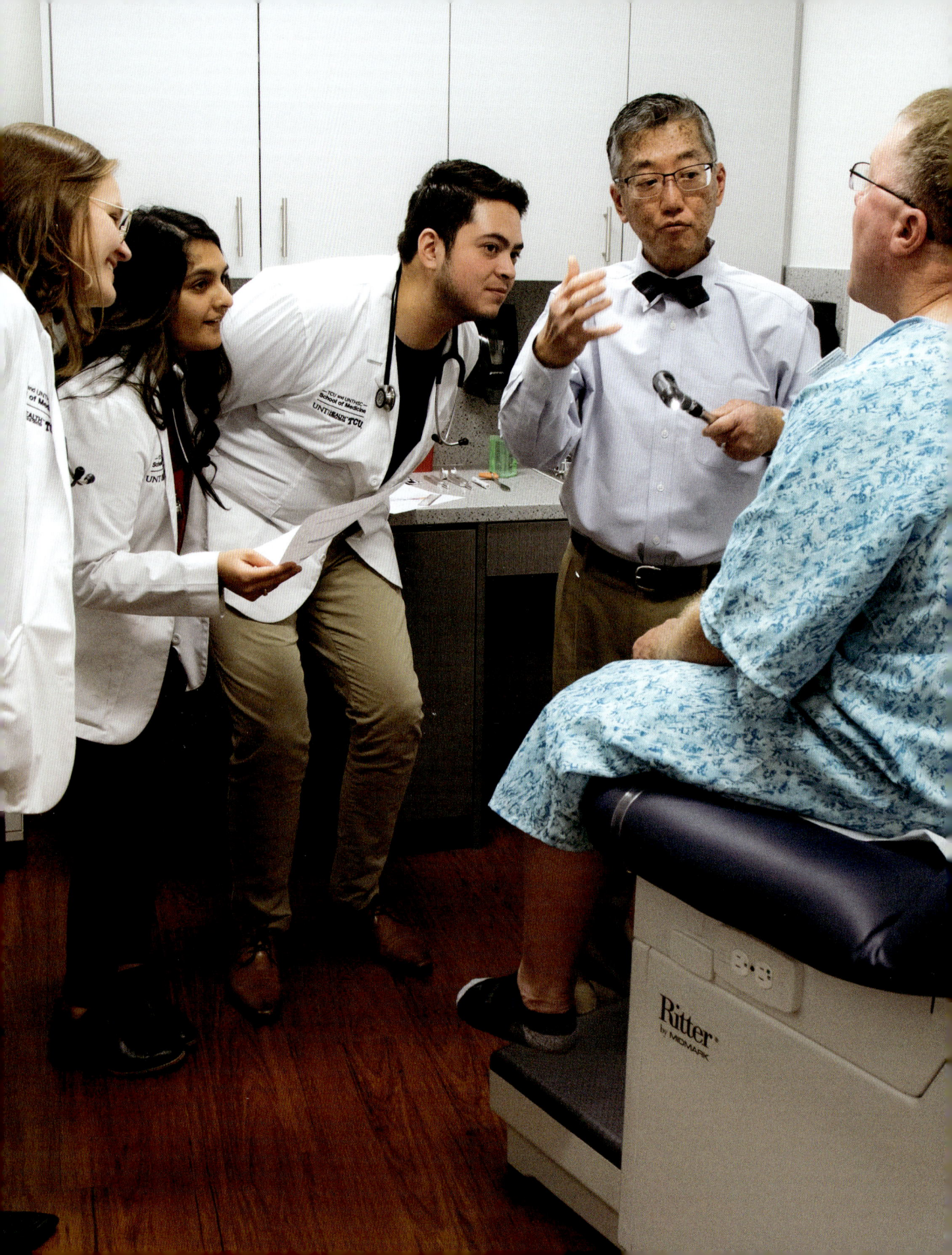

Educating a New Kind of Doctor

When the inaugural class of students at the Anne Burnett Marion School of Medicine first set foot on the TCU campus in July 2019, no one could have predicted that a variant of the SARS-CoV-2 virus would soon upend life around the globe.

That summer, after 23 people died from a racially motivated shooting at a Walmart in El Paso, Texas, gun policies returned to the forefront of political debates. Nine months later, as the pandemic gained traction in the U.S., a Minneapolis police officer murdered George Floyd, sparking worldwide protests and a profound racial reckoning in America.

The medical students were entering a complex time for society and for their profession.

Domestic health care spending grabbed headlines by reaching a record $3.8 trillion. That sum represented 17.7 percent of the U.S. economy, with roughly 60 percent of the medical total going to hospital care, physician and clinical services, and prescription drugs.

In late 2019, Covid-19 originated in Wuhan, China. The U.S. declared a public health emergency on Jan. 31, 2020. Four weeks later, public health officials announced the first death from a laboratory-confirmed case of Covid-19 in the United States.

The World Health Organization declared Covid to be a global pandemic on March 11, 2020. Within weeks, mandatory lockdowns impacted life in the U.S. from coast to coast. Schools, including TCU, pivoted to virtual instruction for the rest of the academic year.

* * *

Two hours after grabbing a breakfast burrito in early March 2020, Jonas Kruse removed the top of a skull. He and his classmates were studying neurology, among the most challenging disciplines medical students encounter during their first year.

Despite the chilly temperature inside the cadaver lab, Kruse brought intensity and focus to the task. His hands did not shake. His stomach never quavered.

"That night I was thinking how I took a brain out of a human head at 9:30 a.m., and it was sort of business as usual," Kruse said. "It's surprising what you can actually get accustomed to."

Edmundo Esparza experienced a range of thoughts and emotions during that first encounter with his cadaver, a 70-something-year-old male who had died of kidney failure. "The body felt very stiff," he said. "I don't know why, but I always expected it to feel more natural."

To everyone's surprise and chagrin, the day the students removed the brains turned out to be the last time they'd see their cadavers. The Covid-19 pandemic meant that after spring break, the inaugural class did not come together again during that first year.

But thanks to the pioneering curriculum high-

Shelby Wildish, left, and fellow medical students Juhi Shah and Edmundo Esparza followed Dr. Song Lee's guidance in examining Chris Clark, one of dozens of actors the medical school employed to portray patients.

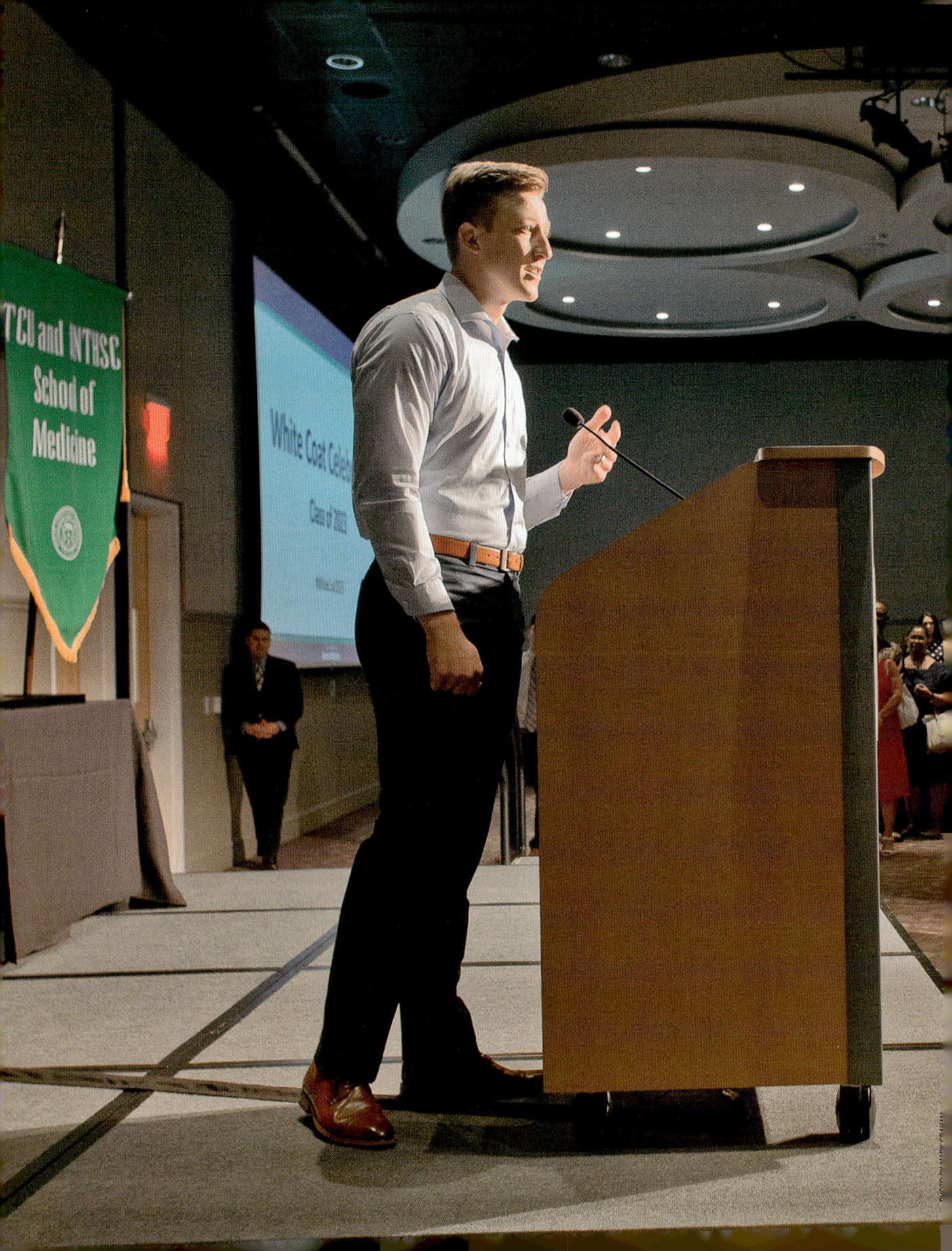

lighting empathy and communication, the school was poised to address student needs while propelling their medical education forward, said the school's founding dean, Dr. Stuart D. Flynn. The pivot to an online-only curriculum enabled the students to maintain an intense pace that kept them on track to becoming doctors in May 2023.

* * *

Eight months earlier, Kruse stood on a stage in TCU's Brown-Lupton University Union, the slight flush on his cheeks more from excitement than nerves. In the audience were his wife, Anabel, as well as his parents and stepparents, who had flown in from Southern California. The Class of 2023 and the faculty had chosen him to deliver a speech during the white coat ceremony, a rite of passage for most new health care students in the U.S.

"It's truly humbling to think about how much has been invested in us," Kruse said as the ballroom thrummed with the energy of his fellow students alongside their families and friends. "It took an army of individuals to get us here, and we're all really excited to be a part of this cutting-edge school."

Flynn, who'd taught surgery and molecular pathology at Yale University before becoming the founding dean of the University of Arizona College of Medicine–Phoenix, nodded to Kruse as the medical student exited the stage and went to stand beside fellow first-year Quinn Losefsky. A few minutes earlier, she'd enjoyed her own moment at the podium while helping to honor entrepreneur H. Paul Dorman. His generous gift of tuition for the entire class's first year of medical school amounted

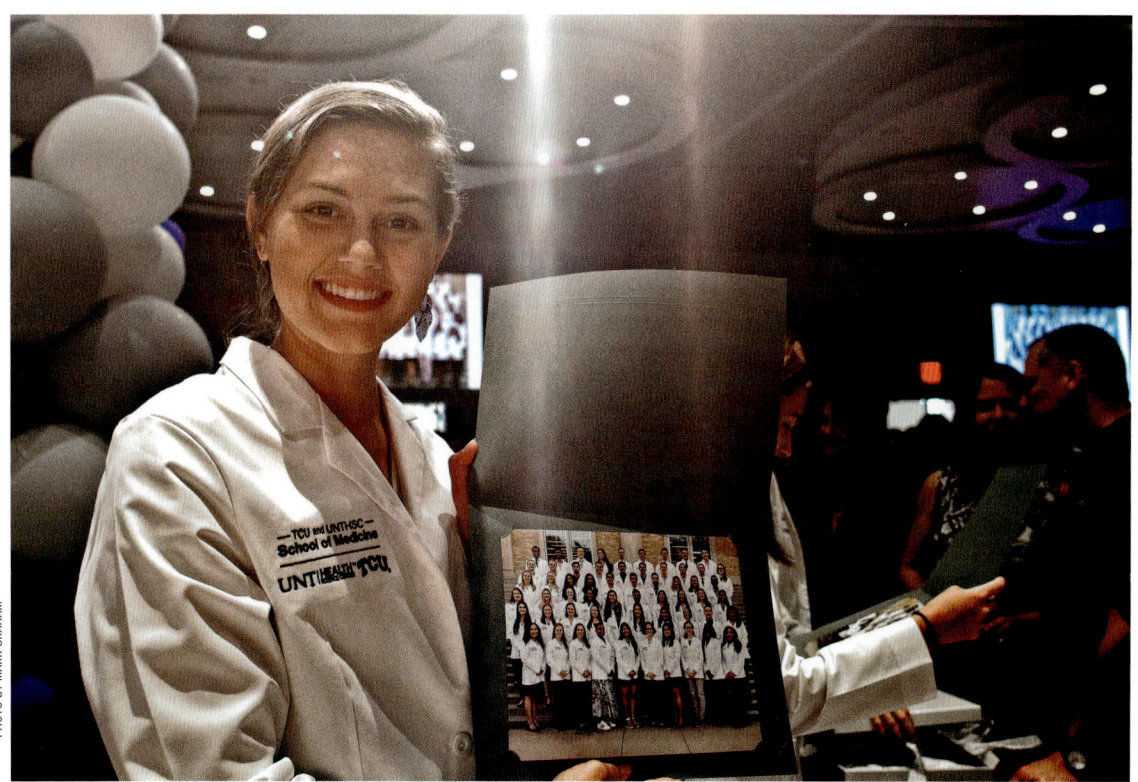

PHOTO BY MARK GRAHAM

Above: Quinn Losefsky and her classmates received a group photo during the white coat celebration, a traditional welcome to medical school for students around the U.S. **Left:** Students in the Class of 2023 elected Jonas Kruse to speak on their behalf at the ceremony, which took place in TCU's Brown-Lupton University Union not long after the start of the first year of medical school.

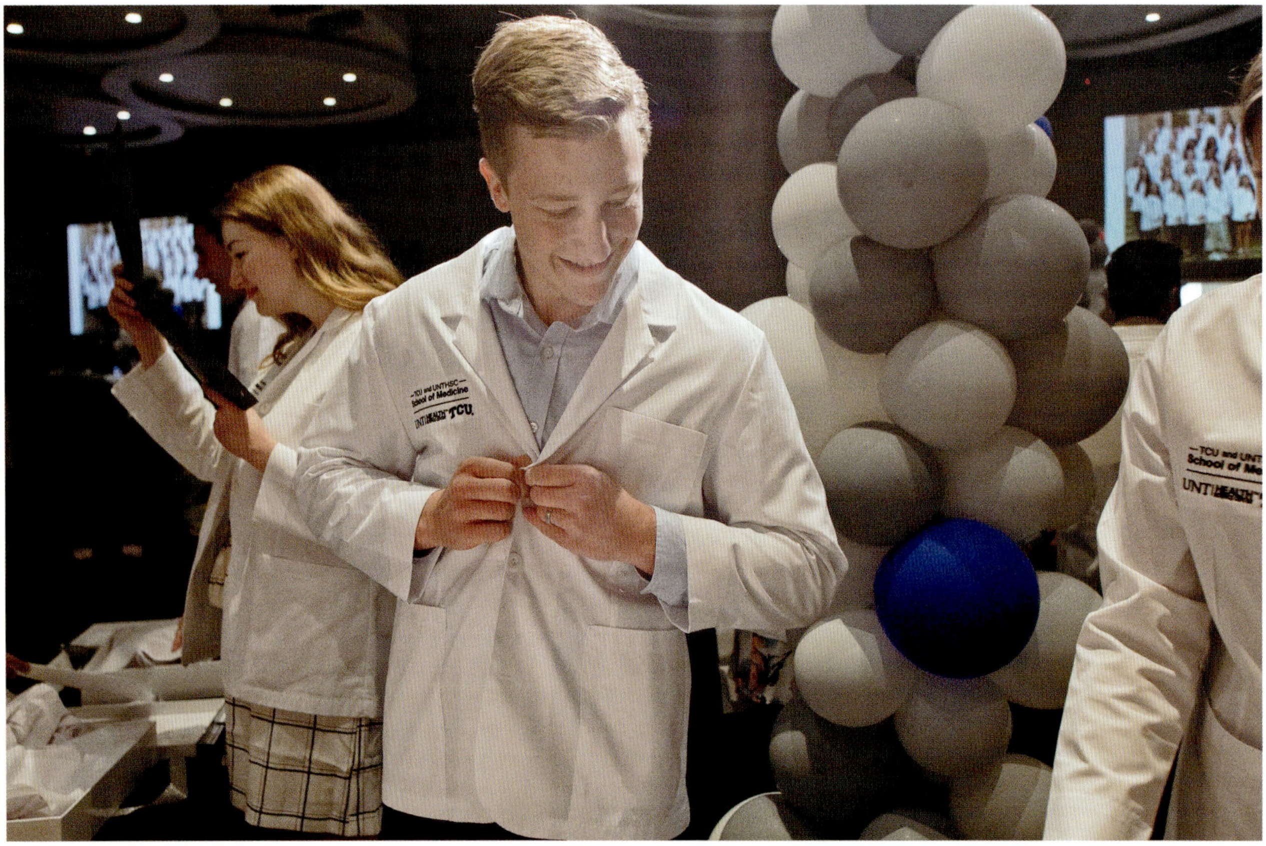

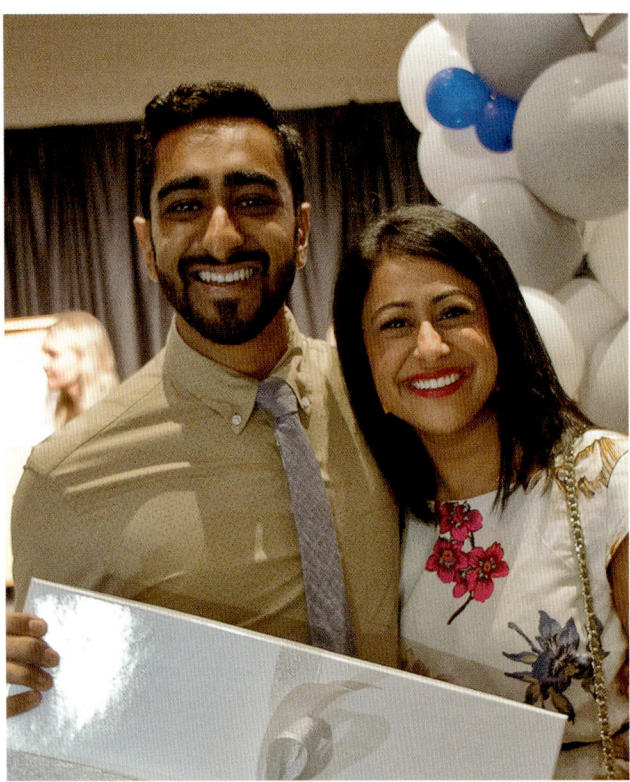

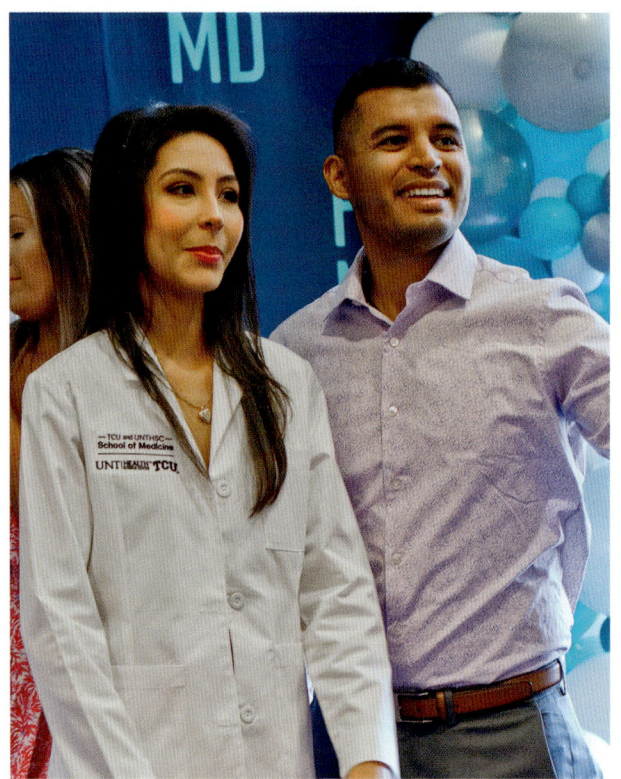

"We all feel like pioneers here. It's an exciting feeling to go somewhere brand new."

Quinn Losefsky

Clockwise from top:

All 60 students in the medical school's inaugural class received white coats and other gifts to mark the beginning of their medical education.

Ive Avila and her husband, Sam, were joined by members of her family who traveled to Fort Worth to support her during the festivities.

Dilan Shah's sister joined him to celebrate the milestone white coat celebration.

to $57,500 per student.

"I understand the need for exceptionally trained physicians," Dorman said, adding that he believed the startup medical school team was "creating the right formula to prepare students in the practice of medicine in the future."

After the speeches, the students were told it was time to untie the silver ribbons on the shirt boxes on tables in front of them. The vibe instantly felt more kid on Christmas morning than serious scholar at one of the most august occasions of their lives. Around the room, students began to shrug on their new white lab coats to tears, gasps and high-fives from those who'd traveled from all over the country to support them.

"We all feel like pioneers here," said Losefsky, who'd earned her undergraduate degree from TCU two months earlier. "It's an exciting feeling to go somewhere brand new."

The lab coat represented the realization of a dream she'd held tight since her early teen years. When the eighth-grade science class at her STEM school in Austin, Texas, dissected a cat, no one else in her group would even touch it. The teacher saw what she'd done and declared it the best dissection he had ever seen.

"That was when I knew I was going to be a surgeon," Losefsky said.

Charna Kinard, who graduated from Loyola University in Chicago, also entered medical school with the goal of becoming a surgeon. She first began considering a career in medicine at age 11, when she lost a grandmother to mesothelioma, a type of lung cancer related to asbestos.

Both Ive Avila, a college classmate of Kinard, and Edmundo Esparza, a University of Texas at El Paso graduate, earned MBAs before embarking on medical school.

Like several of his older siblings, Esparza underperformed as a middle school student, cutting class and causing trouble. He was on the verge of flunking out when a teacher gave him a copy of the first Harry Potter book.

As he tore through the series the summer before high school, Esparza kept asking himself why he was acting out. He identified with the main characters as they demonstrated intelligence and resilience by overcoming odds time and time again. He also delighted in the relationships between the young wizards and the staff at their school, Hogwarts.

"I was just being dumb, ditching with friends," Esparza said, "but I liked school."

Well, maybe not learning about kidneys. Few of the medical students seemed enamored with the study of nephrology, but

Esparza found the experience no less than painful. His father's Type 2 diabetes had gone unmanaged for years. Mundo Esparza developed diabetic neuropathy, which his son described as damage to the nerves resulting from unchecked high blood sugar. That in turn forced him on dialysis.

"Everything spun off the diabetes," Esparza said. His father's kidneys stopped working. His brain and heart suffered, too.

The elder Esparza had served in the Mexican state police, making him eligible for care at a state hospital just over the El Paso border. But there he was misdiagnosed. The byzantine health care system in Mexico also meant that doctors there could deal only with the presenting symptom. So when he went to the hospital for heart palpitations, his medical team looked at nothing beyond that. When he developed an infection in the hospital, they had to discharge him for the heart problem before readmitting him for the new infection, a process that could take anywhere from hours to days.

"These things are so easily taken care of here if you have the money," Esparza said. "There was no reason for the progression, let alone the outcome."

The family buried Mundo Esparza on March 1, 2018. His youngest child started medical school 494 days later.

* * *

Dilan Shah began medical school not long after attending a two-week silent meditation retreat on the Indonesian island of Java. The experience amplified his belief that he could help people manage their emotions at a time when the National Institute

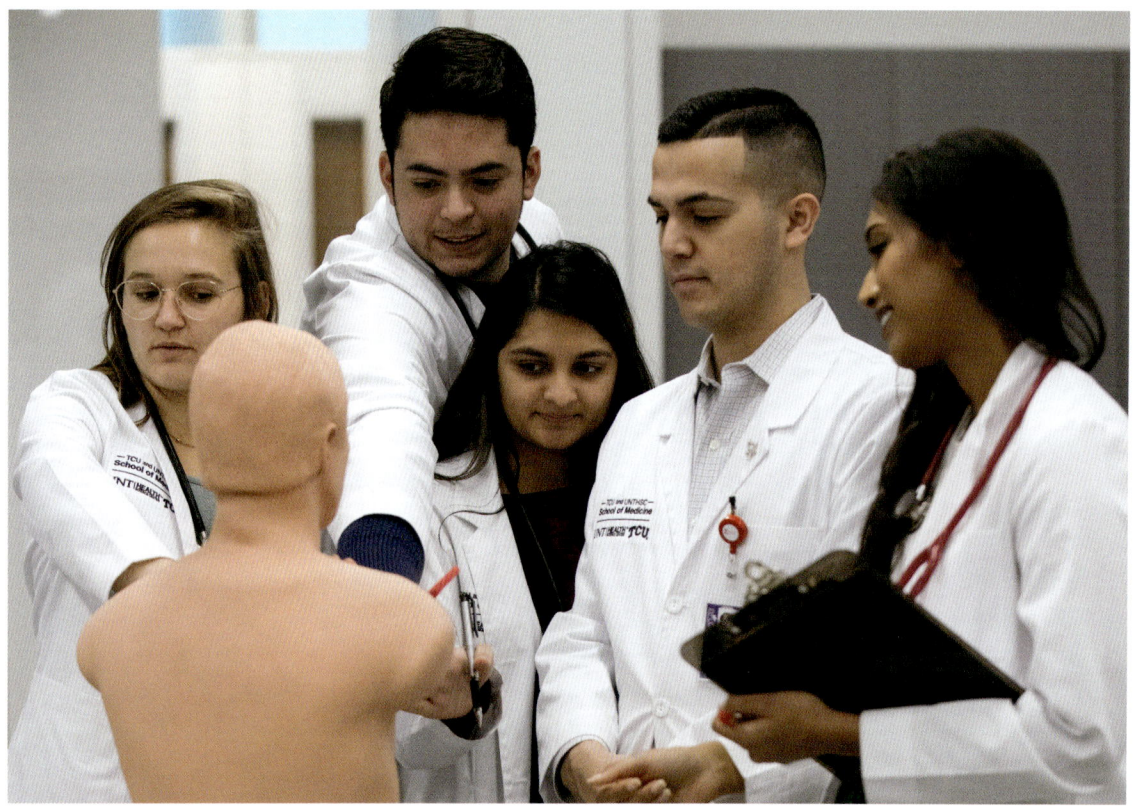

Above, from left: Shelby Wildish, Esparza, Juhi Shah, Connor Rodriguez and Hira Nazim listened to heartbeat patterns in a simulation classroom. Right: Esparza armed himself with information before entering a simulated patient room to conduct an exam.

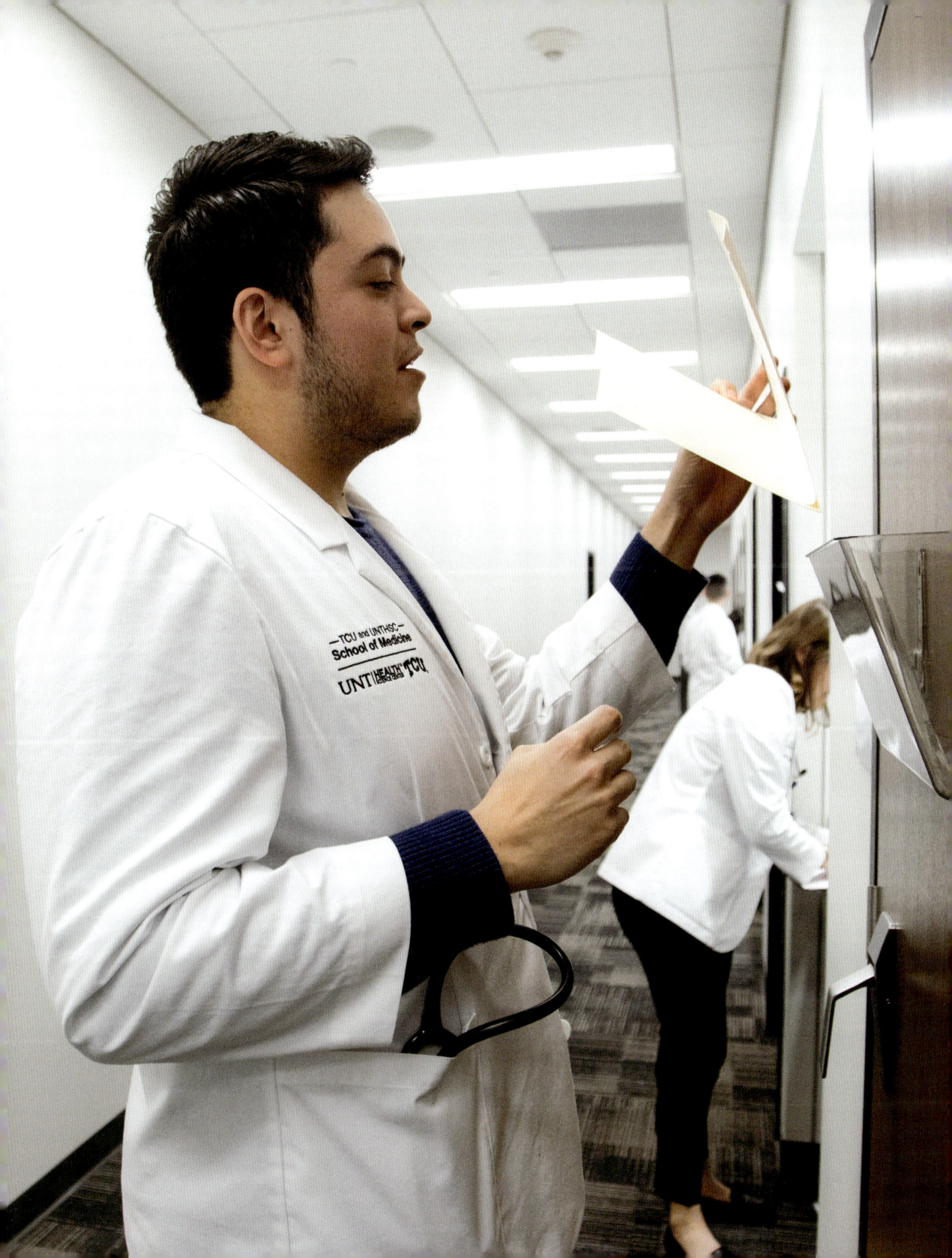

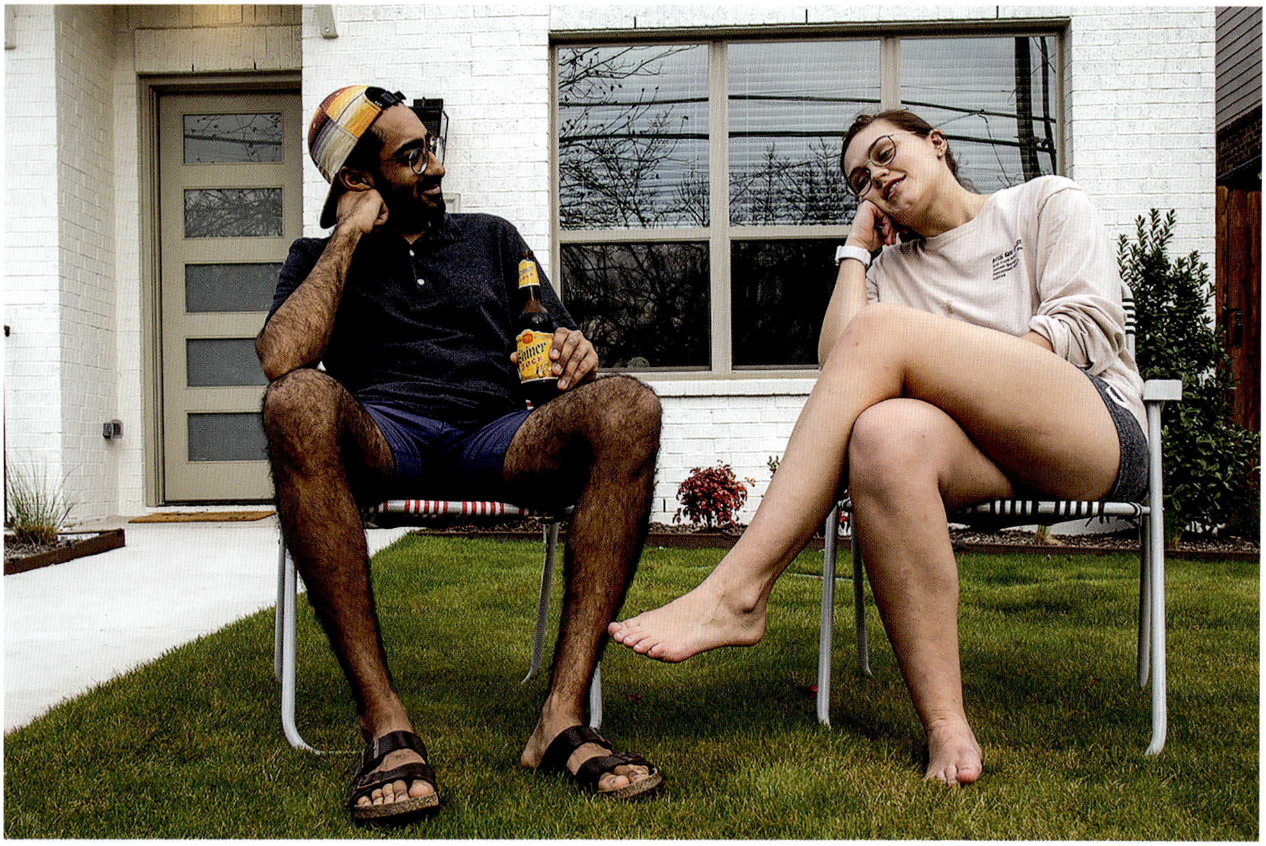

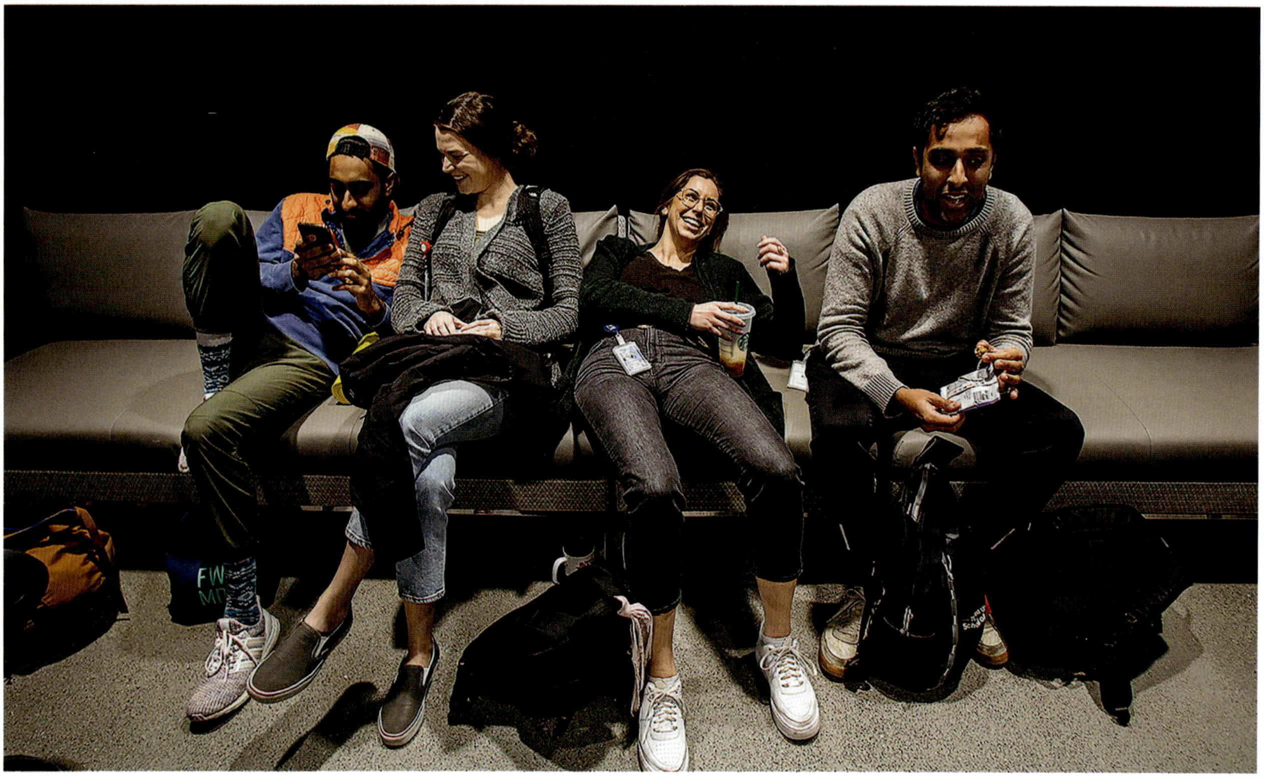

PHOTOS BY MARK GRAHAM

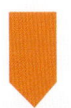

"For so many years, I'd been told you can't wear your feelings on your sleeve to be a doctor, that you have to have distance between the patient. But the storytelling and small groups we have at this school give us the chance to see that's wrong."

Charna Kinard

Top: Shah and Losefsky relaxed at the townhouse they shared. Having a built-in study partner helped Losefsky weather the transition to stay-at-home learning, she said.

Bottom: Shah, Kathryn Biddle, McKenna Chalman and Sameer Allahabadi enjoyed a moment of downtime during the busy weeks of their first year of medical education.

of Mental Health reported rising rates of depression and other emotional disorders.

The increase disproportionately impacted health care professionals, particularly those in training. The American Medical Association reported in 2019 that medical students were "three times likelier to die of suicide than their counterparts in the general population."

Shah and the rest of his class were introduced to the Compassionate Practice® within days of starting medical school. Throughout the year, they received diversity training with an emphasis on microaggressions and how biases in race, gender and sexuality can impact health care. The medical school's staff worked with students on improvisational, role-playing and storytelling techniques typical of a theater curriculum, with the goal of improving health communication and empathy.

In monthly written reflections, the students explored how they felt about patients and classes. "We can use it as a way to talk through the anxieties we have felt when we've asked a patient about something really personal," Esparza said. "It's part of learning how to deal with the responsibility that comes with being a doctor."

In other assigned writings, students took the perspective of a patient to help increase their sensitivity. "For so many years, I'd been told you can't wear your feelings on your sleeve to be a doctor, that you have to have distance between the patient," Kinard said. "But the storytelling and small groups we have at this school give us the chance to see that's wrong."

To de-emphasize competition and encourage collaboration, the medical school made its classes pass-fail while rejecting traditional ranking systems. "It only serves to hurt the collective if someone else is struggling," said Kruse, who noted that during the first semester he received daily texts from fellow students asking questions or sharing resources.

"There are no classic gunners here, the kind of med student obsessed with being No. 1," Losefsky said. "We don't have a No. 1."

* * *

In response to the Covid-19 pandemic, TCU, like most educational institutions, moved instruction to the virtual realm. The initial announcement of the suspension of in-person classes came toward the end of spring break.

To blow off steam after an intense winter that included physics-laden pulmonology, Kruse, Shah and six other students traveled together to Southern California, where they spent time at Disneyland and the beach. The group of guys devoted most mornings of their vacation to reviewing online flashcards and medical terminology.

Avila, who owns a ranch near Austin with her husband, Sam, joined him on a road trip around Texas in their fifth wheel, a type of RV pulled by another vehicle. During her first year of medical school, she saved rent money by living in the camper.

At the end of spring break and after much consideration about how best to manage her studies, Avila returned to Fort Worth with her dogs, Winter and Blue. But within weeks of that difficult decision, her husband's medical recruiting job went remote because of Covid. The couple moved their farm animals to her parents' nearby ranch before he joined her permanently in Fort Worth.

"In some ways the pandemic was good for us as a couple," she said.

Kinard was returning from a conference in Kentucky when she learned that in-person instruction would be delayed. For months afterward, she struggled to process the implications of the public health crisis. Keeping up with endless news cycles while diving back into her studies — particularly demanding neurology — felt overwhelming, she said.

Like most of her classmates, Kinard longed for a return to normalcy. A gamer who competed in tournaments, both solo and with a team, she'd weighed a professional gaming career before applying to medical school. As a TCU medical student, she regularly played cards with her classmates and cheered on their pingpong tournaments. Then the pandemic upended life for everyone.

During the city's safer-at-home directive, Kinard spent most of her days alone in her apartment, wondering whether she should return to Chicago.

"It was never in my plan for med school to study at home," she said.

Losefsky believed she fared well both emotionally

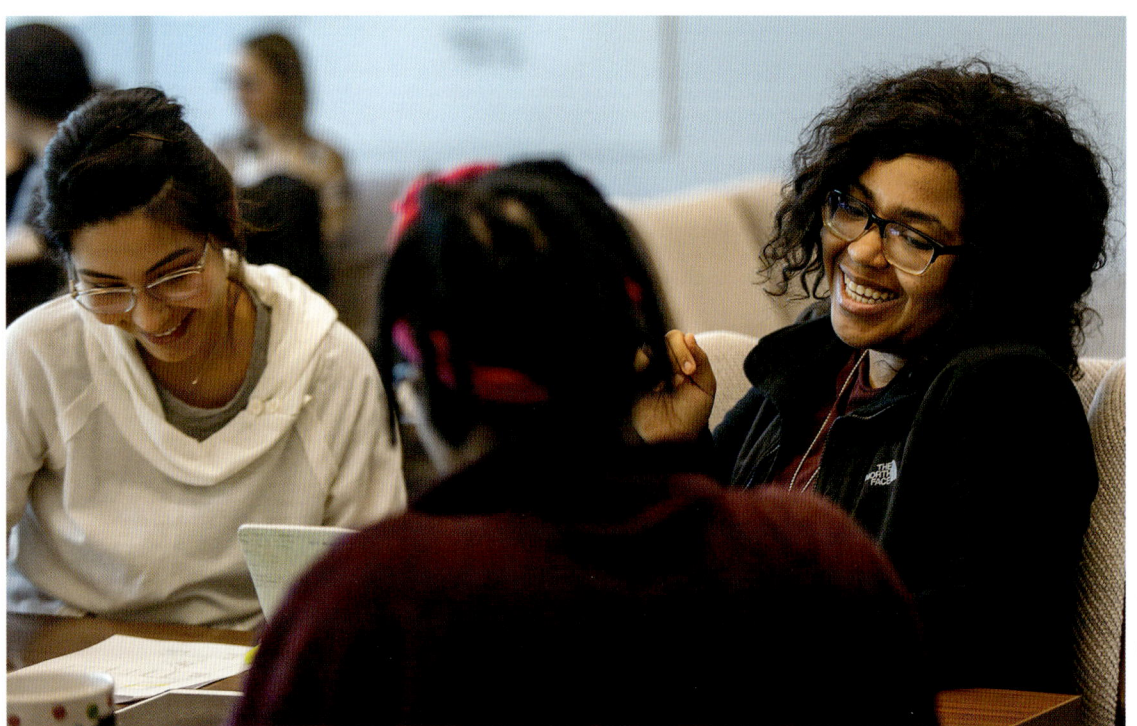

PHOTO BY MARK GRAHAM

Above: Avila, left, and Kinard tackled work in pulmonology, a discipline many of the students found challenging. Right: Avila's beloved rescue dogs Winter, left, and Blue helped her relieve stress throughout medical school.

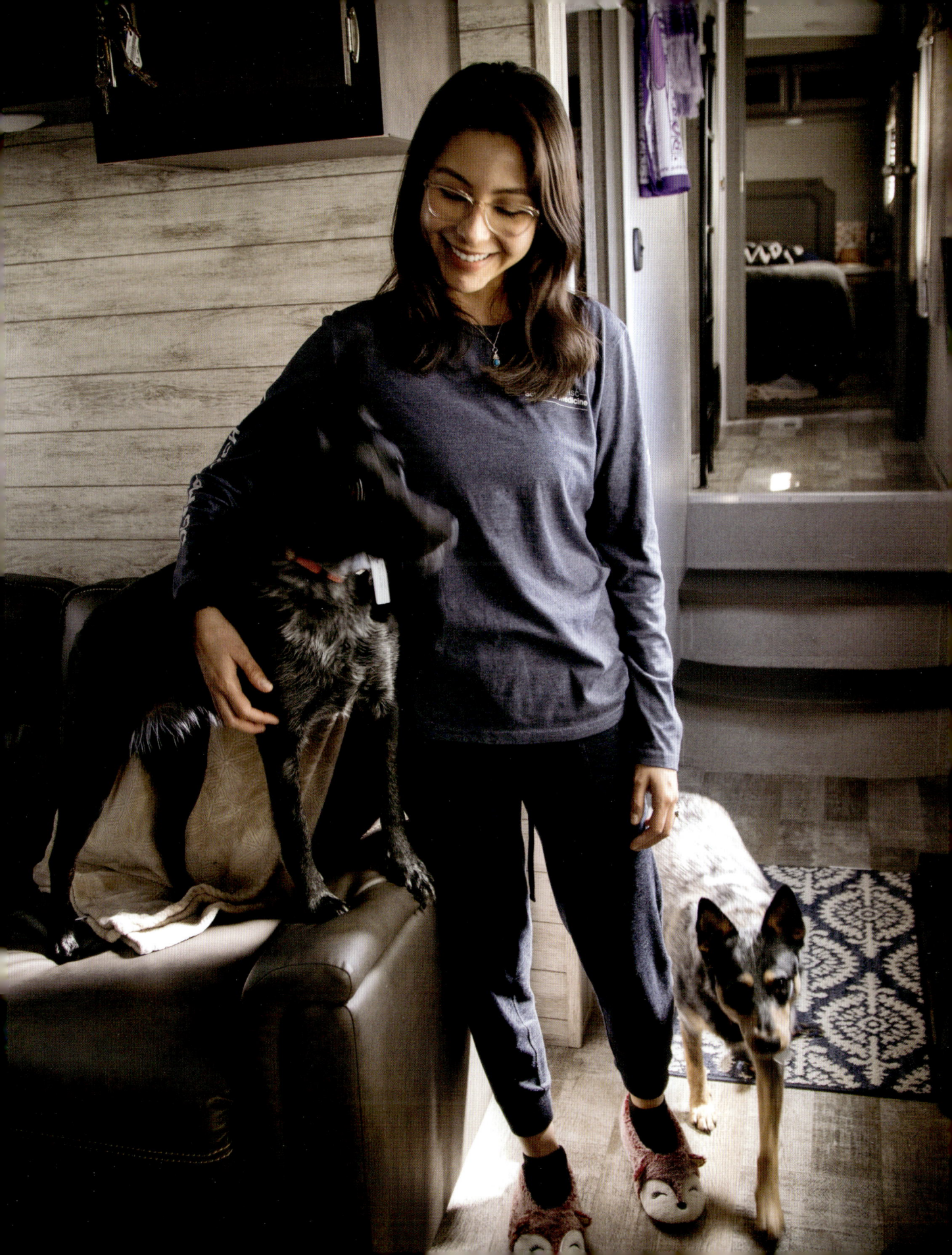

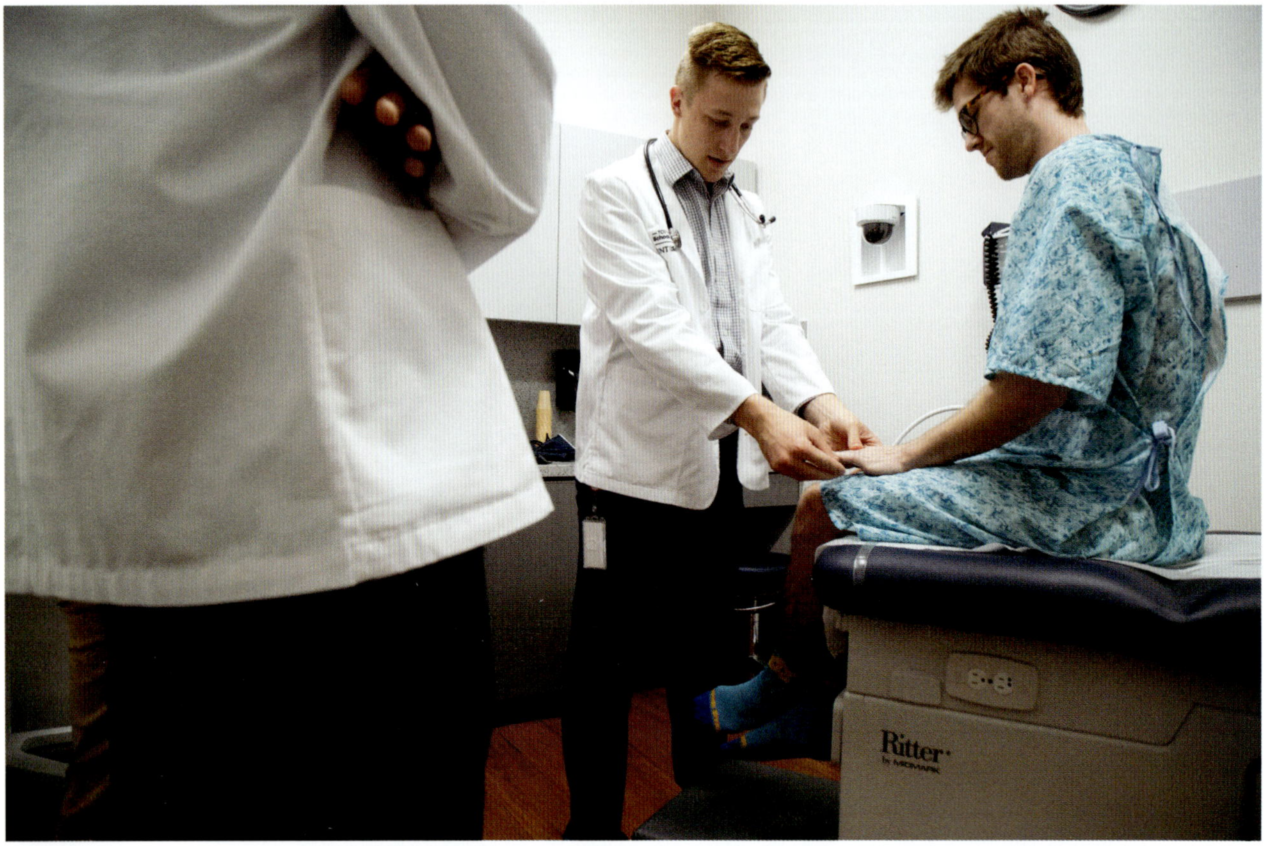
Ritter

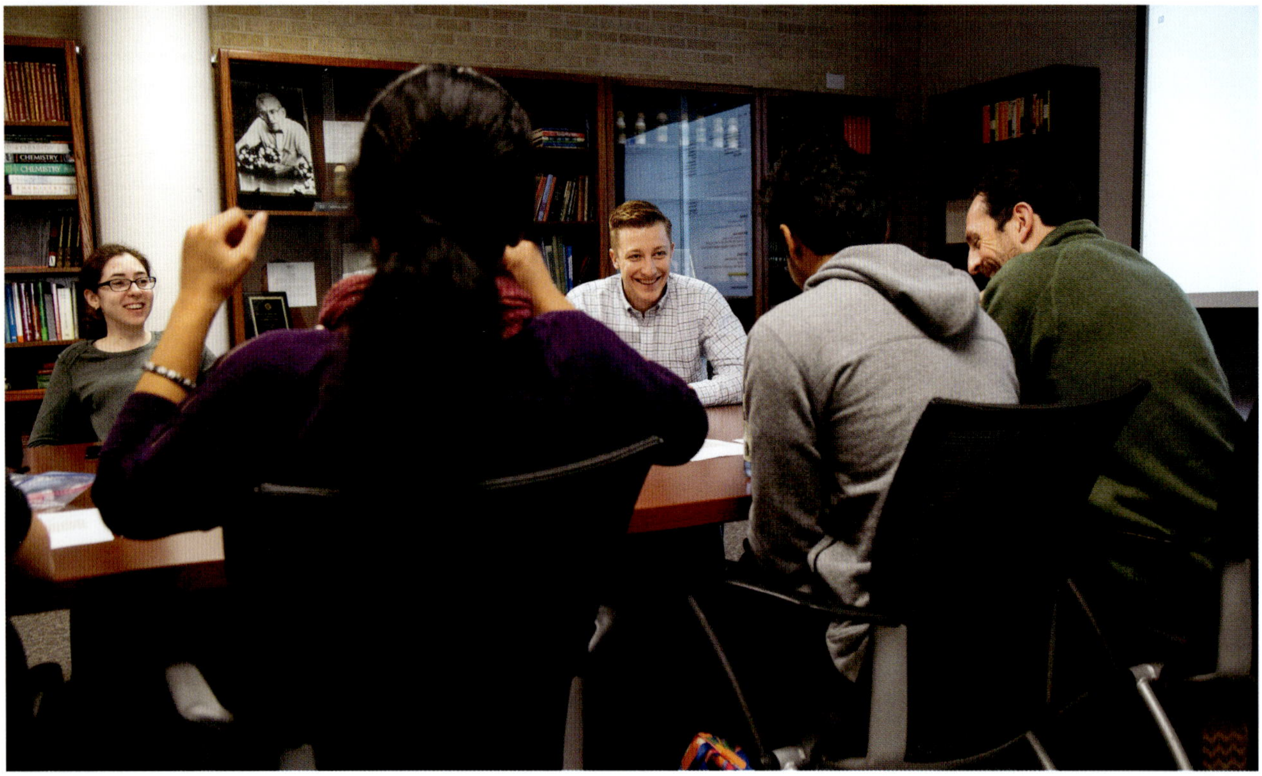
CHEMISTRY
CHEMISTRY

> "Whenever I start to think about how expensive the school is, I look around and remind myself there are always at least five doctors near us."

Dilan Shah

Top: Interactive classes are a hallmark of TCU's School of Medicine. Kruse asked patient-actor Michael Carver-Simmons to describe his symptoms and medical concerns while he conducted a physical exam.

Bottom: During the first year, small groups, including Kruse's, received a patient case each Monday. By Friday, they were expected to have an accurate diagnosis and to have created an effective treatment plan.

and academically during the pandemic thanks in large part to her built-in study partner. She and Shah started medical school as strangers and clicked right away. In December 2019, Shah and his parents purchased a townhouse for him in a northwestern suburb of Fort Worth. Losefsky moved into a spare bedroom weeks later, right as the pandemic began ravaging Italy.

The rest of the spring, the lifelong athlete tweaked her routine, which no longer included the gym, library and coffee shops. "I'm always reevaluating what works for me," Losefsky said. "I love med school and don't ever want to burn out."

Shah credited the tools he entered medical school with for helping him cope with the pandemic. The Austin College graduate practices Vipassana, a form of meditation that he describes as accepting one's reality — anxiety, fear and all. Mediating under his favorite tree near the Trinity River made him feel centered and focused, with a renewed sense of calm.

Esparza felt a surge of angst when the school announced it would remain online-only through the rest of the 2019-20 academic year. He shared an apartment with the same two classmates, Alex Tolman and Hermenegildo Charrez-Baxcajay, all four years at TCU and made it a point to become more engaged with online classes as the pandemic raged.

The medical school's transition to virtual instruction did go relatively smoothly in part because independent learning in a team setting resides in the school's DNA. But that didn't mean connecting online was always easy. "When we're working together on Zoom," Kinard said, "people are much quicker to shut someone down or dismiss them.

"The goal was always to raise each other up, but I do feel the distance has taken away some of the common considerations we would give each other in person," she said.

From the desk she ordered for her apartment when the school libraries closed, Kinard joined classmates online for courses such as Patient-Centered Inquiry-Based Learning. On Mondays, groups of seven or eight students would receive a patient case that they were expected to solve by Friday.

The small groups met on Zoom in late March 2020 to consider a patient with Bell's palsy, a sudden weakness or paralysis in facial muscles. Students researched symptoms and underlying causes to come up with interventions and recommendations for treatments.

"It's working OK," Kinard said, "but I am finding myself less willing to be vulnerable and ask questions when we're separated digitally."

"The communication is not nearly as rich because we're not together, and our group is definitely more quiet," Kruse said. "But if this had to happen, I'm really grateful it was during our first year instead of later, when nearly everything is clinical."

"The school has done an excellent job of making the curriculum online," Esparza said, "but it's hard to replace being face-to-face with everyone." He believed the isolation took a toll on the connection his classmates had.

"There are things like seeing patients and physical exams on the standardized patients [actors hired to perform as people seeking medical care] that we can't do remotely," Flynn said, "but none of that is career-altering or will impact their residency placement."

* * *

Online classes disrupted more than camaraderie among the classmates. Esparza said he also missed seeing the medical school faculty. The faculty, which includes physicians, scientists and public health professionals, then numbered nearly 450. (That figure would grow to 1,500 by spring 2024.)

"Whenever I start to think about how expensive the school is," Shah said, "I look around and remind myself there are always at least five doctors near us."

Most medical schools split students into small groups, with a new physician interacting with them every week, Flynn said. At the Burnett School of Medicine, students work one-on-one and in small groups all four years with many of the same doctors.

"We don't often say it this way," Flynn noted, "but physicians are teachers."

Faculty members add another layer of emotional support to the student experience. The first week on the TCU campus, the students were divided into six teams. Ten new students join a team each successive year, with two physicians coaching each group.

In the wake of the pandemic, physician-coach Debra Atkisson doubled down on her students' well-

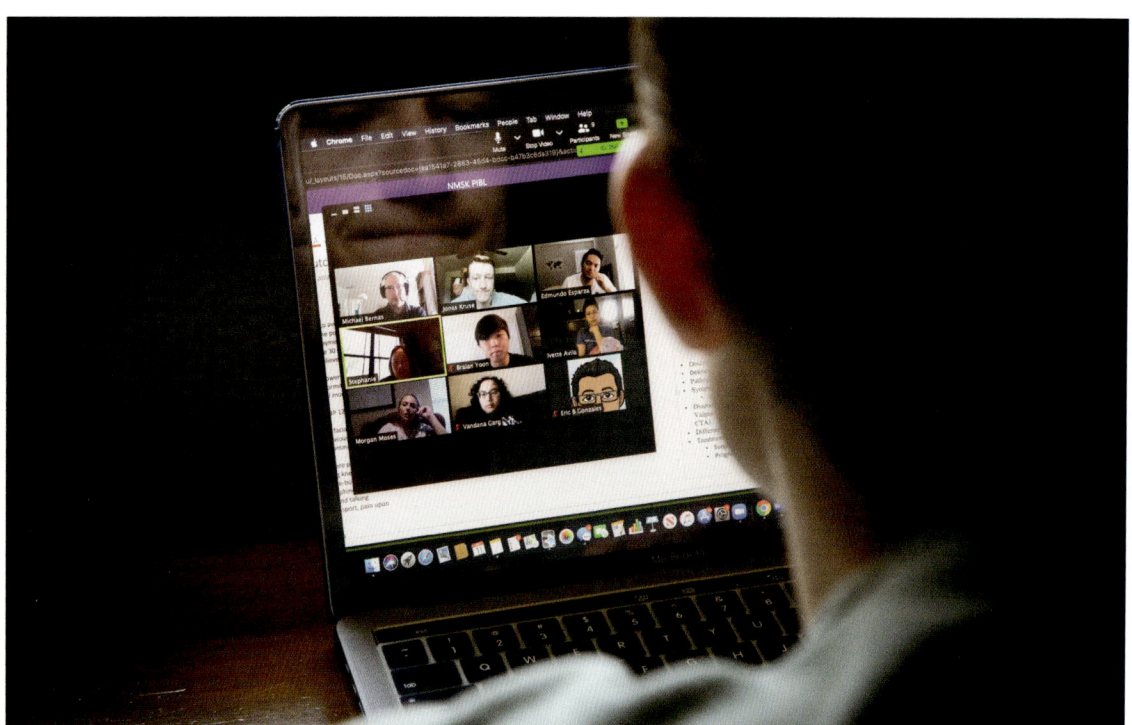

Above: From March to September 2020, all of TCU's medical school classes, including this one that Kruse attended from his Fort Worth home office, went virtual as a result of the pandemic. Right: Kruse and his wife, Anabel, masked up in the fight against Covid-19.

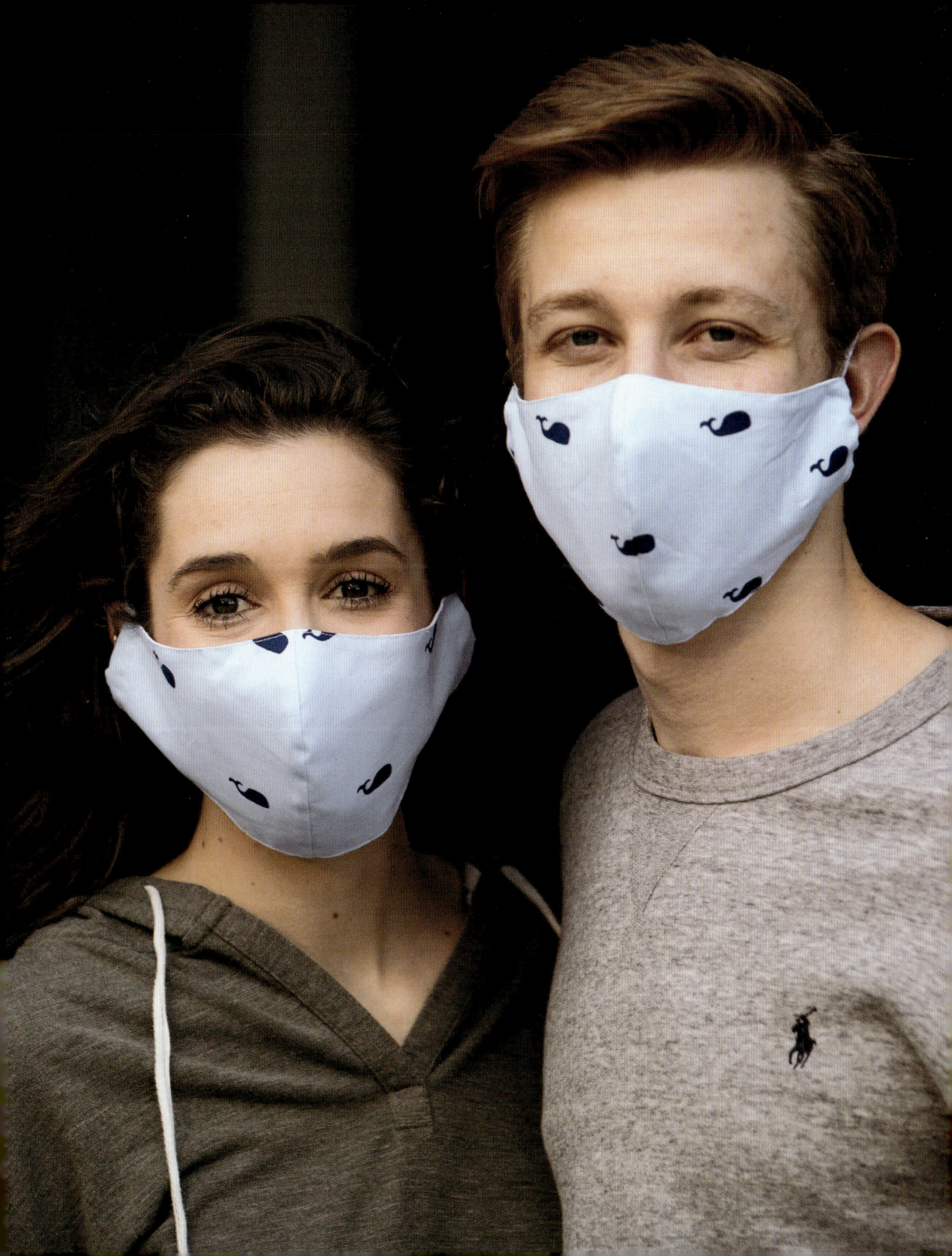

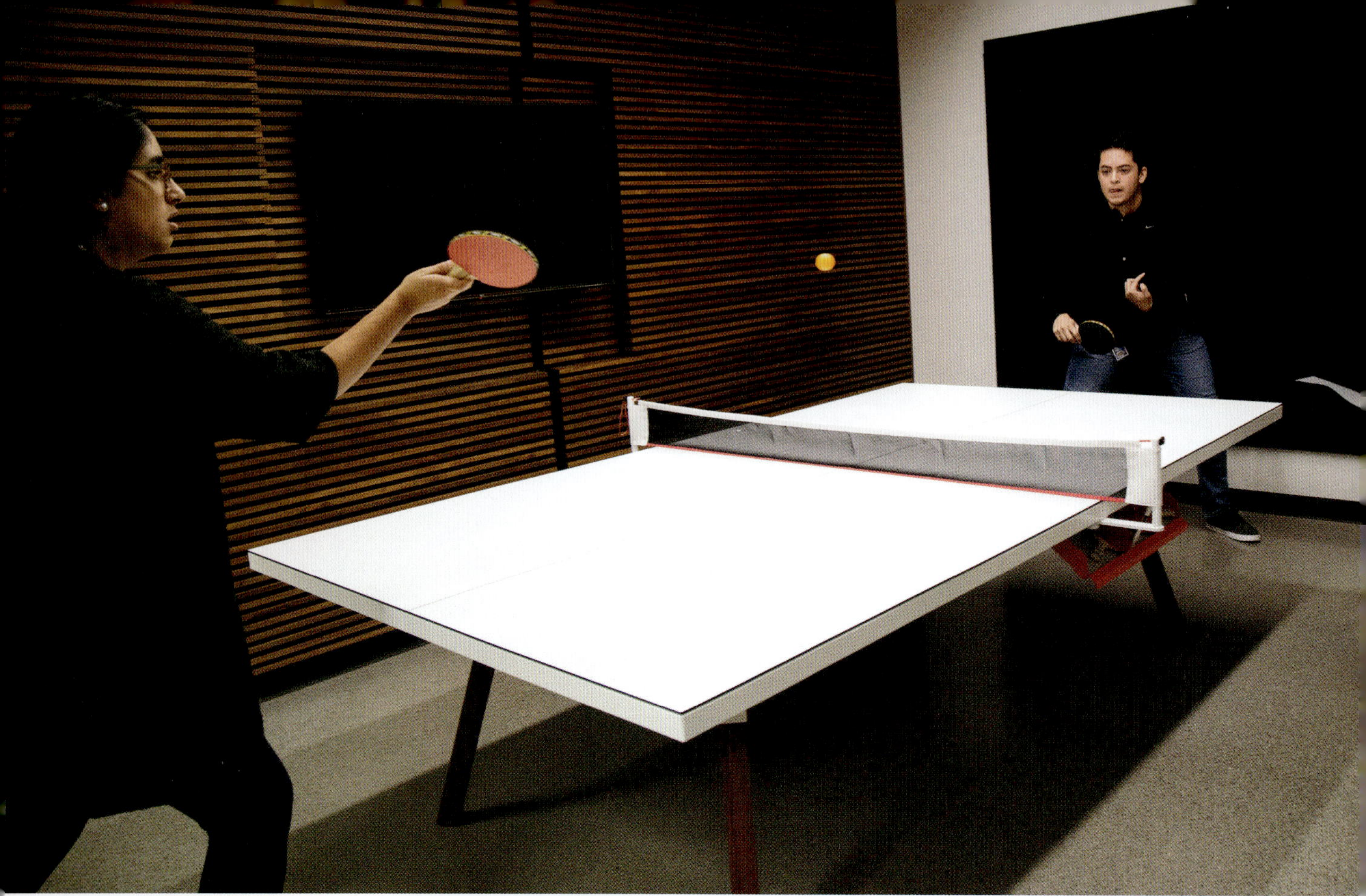

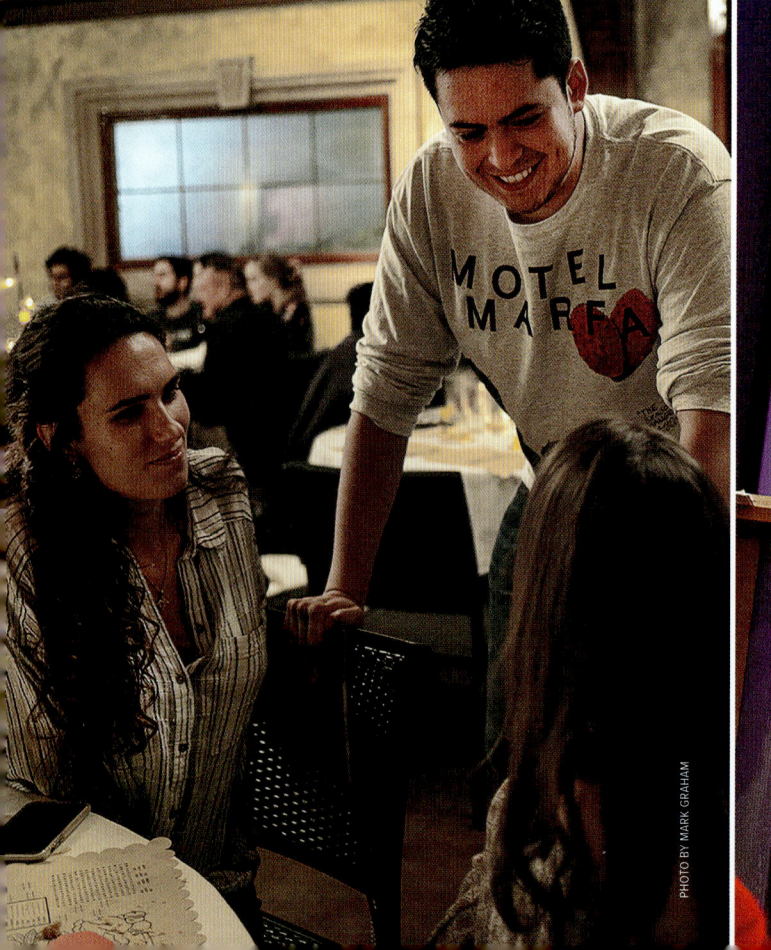

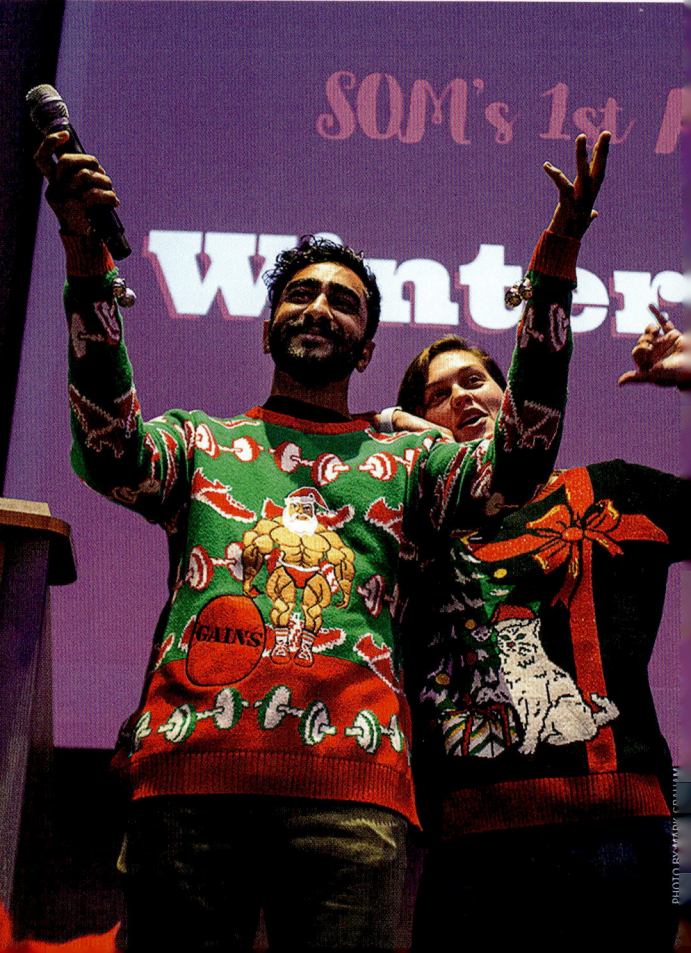

being. The Fort Worth psychiatrist met weekly via Zoom with her team of 10, which included Esparza, Losefsky and Kruse. Atkisson often asked how they were maintaining a sense of normalcy during such an abnormal time. "One of the things the school has done such an amazing job at is working with students on their own awareness of compassion, empathy and whole-person view," she said.

During the first six months of the academic year, Atkisson saw members of her group at frequent social events, such as a Friendsgiving dinner at Joe T. Garcia's and the student-initiated Winterfest. Shah emceed the holiday gathering, which featured student vocal performances, a baking contest and a gift exchange.

Esparza became especially close to Atkisson ("She can crack me like an egg!"). He sought her out in February 2020 to discuss what he saw as a growing problem with focus. "I wait for the anxiety and the thrill of test week to come around," he said, "and I don't want to rely on that anymore."

* * *

The pandemic also meant the school had to pause the students' clinical rotations, which had been a big draw for Kinard, who gave up a spot at Dartmouth University's medical school when she was admitted from the Burnett waitlist. She and the rest of her classmates gambled on an institution with neither a reputation nor a track record largely because of its intention to approach medical school differently.

Most medical students attend traditional lectures for hours a day, especially the first year. None of the classes at this medical school is in a lecture format. In addition, every student works with patients under the supervision of physicians all four years, another hallmark. Some medical schools, such as Harvard University's, offer similar

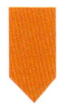

"The patient must be at the center of everything we do every day, which is easy to say and very difficult to execute."

Dr. Mohanakrishnan Sathyamoorthy

training, but those programs do not begin until the third year and not every student participates.

Early in her first year, Avila began an integrated clerkship at a family medicine clinic in the nearby city of Aledo. A patient she saw in January 2020 told her that he was not doing well. With an upward tilt of his chin and a note of outrage in his voice, Russell Webb announced that between Thanksgiving and Christmas he'd gained weight — far more than the stereotypical 5 pounds. Fifty, maybe 60 pounds, he conceded to Avila as she stood near her preceptor, Dr. Shaun Kretzschmar.

Avila asked Webb if he'd recently changed medications or started taking any new supplements. No, and the arthritis in both shoulders and his numb fingertips weren't getting any better, he said.

Would he consider a steroid injection, Avila asked, steadily holding his gaze.

"I'd rather be shot with a 9 mm than be shot with a needle," he fired back.

Outside the exam room, the family medicine specialist told her that she'd done well with a patient who can be prickly. "I like him," said Avila, who first met Webb in the fall. That wintry day, he was the sixth patient that the doctor and medical student had

Clockwise from top: During the first year of medical school, student leader Esparza helped organize frequent pingpong tournaments with his classmates, including future surgeon Kavneet Kaur; Shah and Losefsky donned ugly sweaters for Winterfest in December 2019; Sophie Wix, Esparza and their classmates celebrated Friendsgiving at Joe T. Garcia's in the Fort Worth Stockyards in November 2019.

seen together in a 90-minute span.

Until the pandemic reached North Texas in March 2020, Kruse, Esparza and Losefsky had spent two afternoons a month at an internal medicine clinic about 20 miles southeast of TCU's main campus. There the students shadowed physicians as part of their training.

Losefsky "came up with things that I didn't expect a first-year student to catch," said Dr. Khuong Phan, who sees around 100 patients a week at Mansfield Medical Associates.

When Losefsky entered the room of Clifford Simmons, he greeted her like a friend or, perhaps, granddaughter, considering their ages. She'd seen him the previous month, on the day before she turned 23.

Losefsky donned purple gloves to examine Simmons' swollen legs and listen to his heart. She excused herself to go tell Phan that she thought Simmons was in atrial fibrillation, one of several types of arrhythmia. In short order, the doctor confirmed her diagnosis.

When the Covid lockdowns put the students' clinical rotations on hold, Losefsky asked Phan if he would send her patient charts to review at home. She pored over the cases, wishing she were back in the exam room.

"The patient must be at the center of everything we do every day, which is easy to say and very difficult to execute," said Dr. Mohanakrishnan Sathyamoorthy. The cardiologist and chair of the school's department of internal medicine praised the inaugural cohort of TCU medical students as "being collaborative, kind-spirited and empathetic. My general impression of this first class is it's a home run."

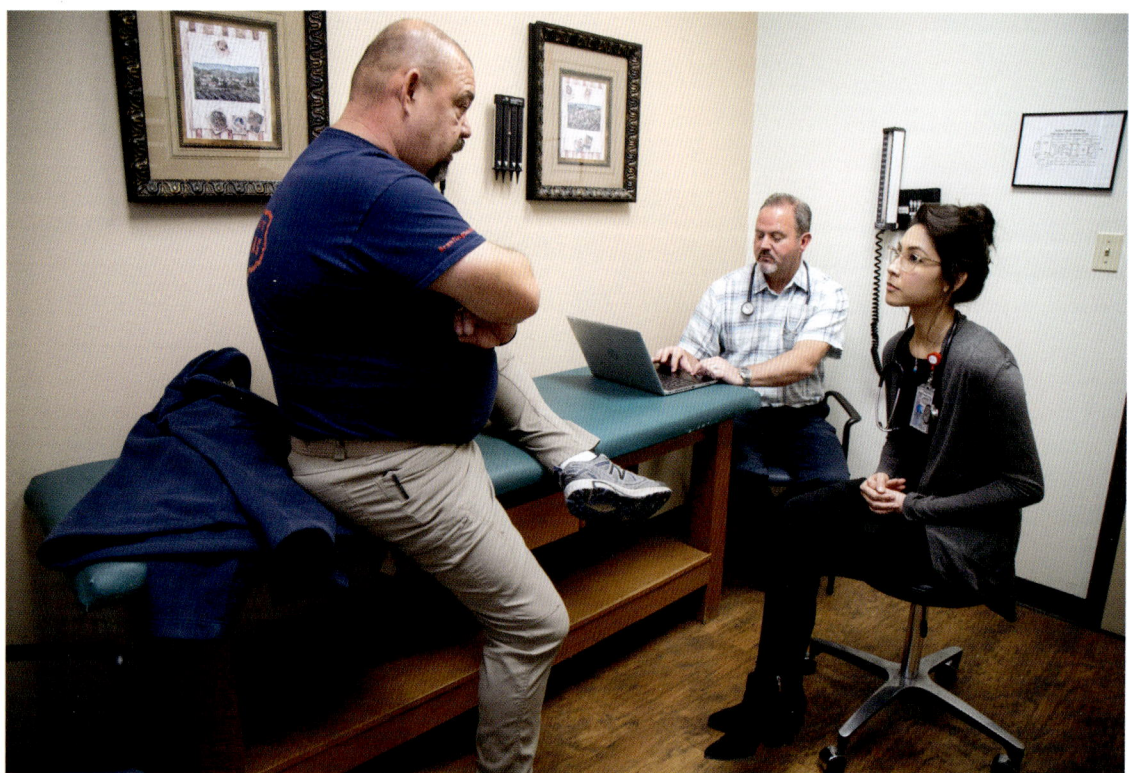

Above and right: Avila spoke with and examined patient Russell Webb under the auspices of Dr. Shaun Kretzschmar, who runs a family practice clinic in Aledo, Texas. TCU's School of Medicine departs from most others in the U.S. in that students work with real patients during their first year.

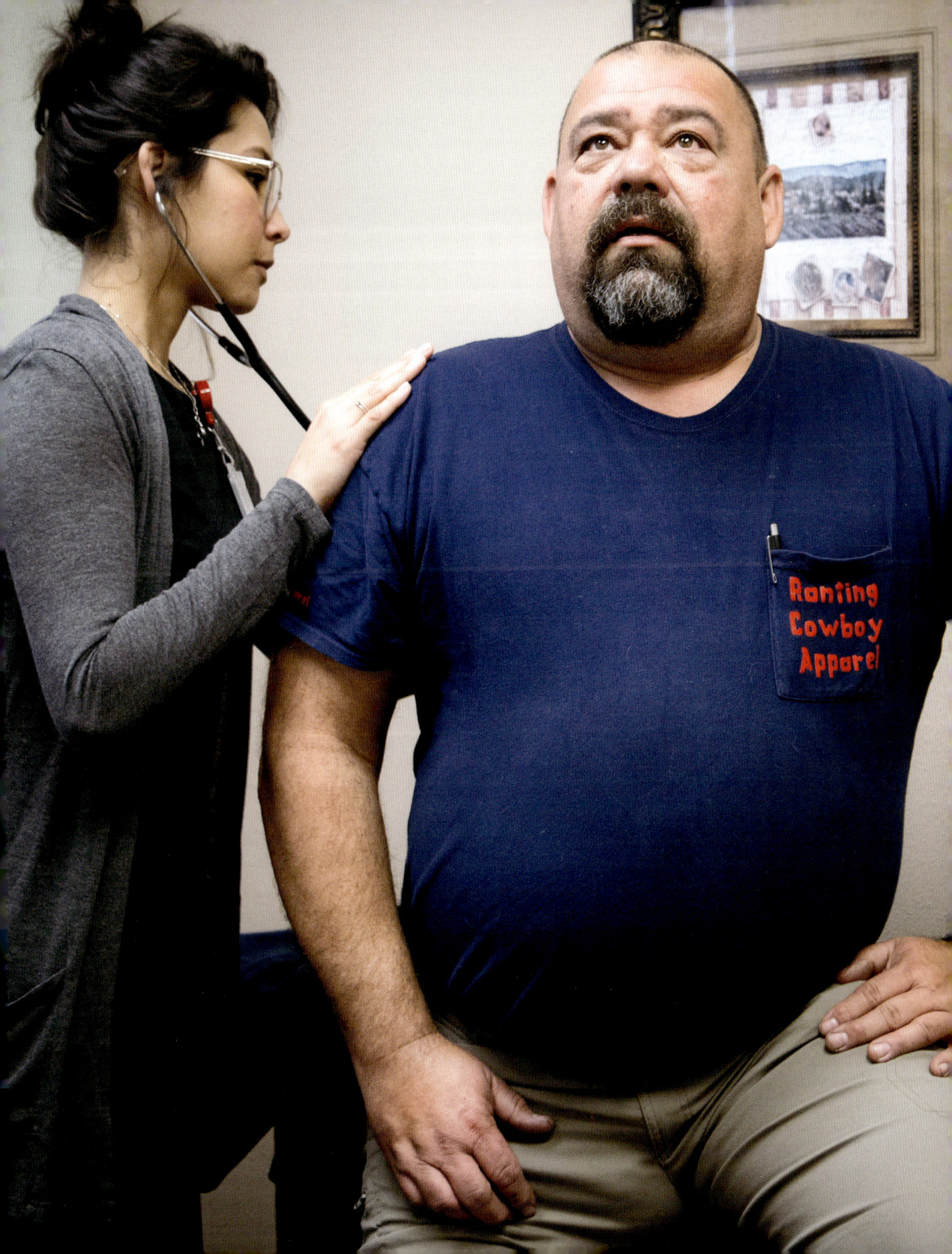

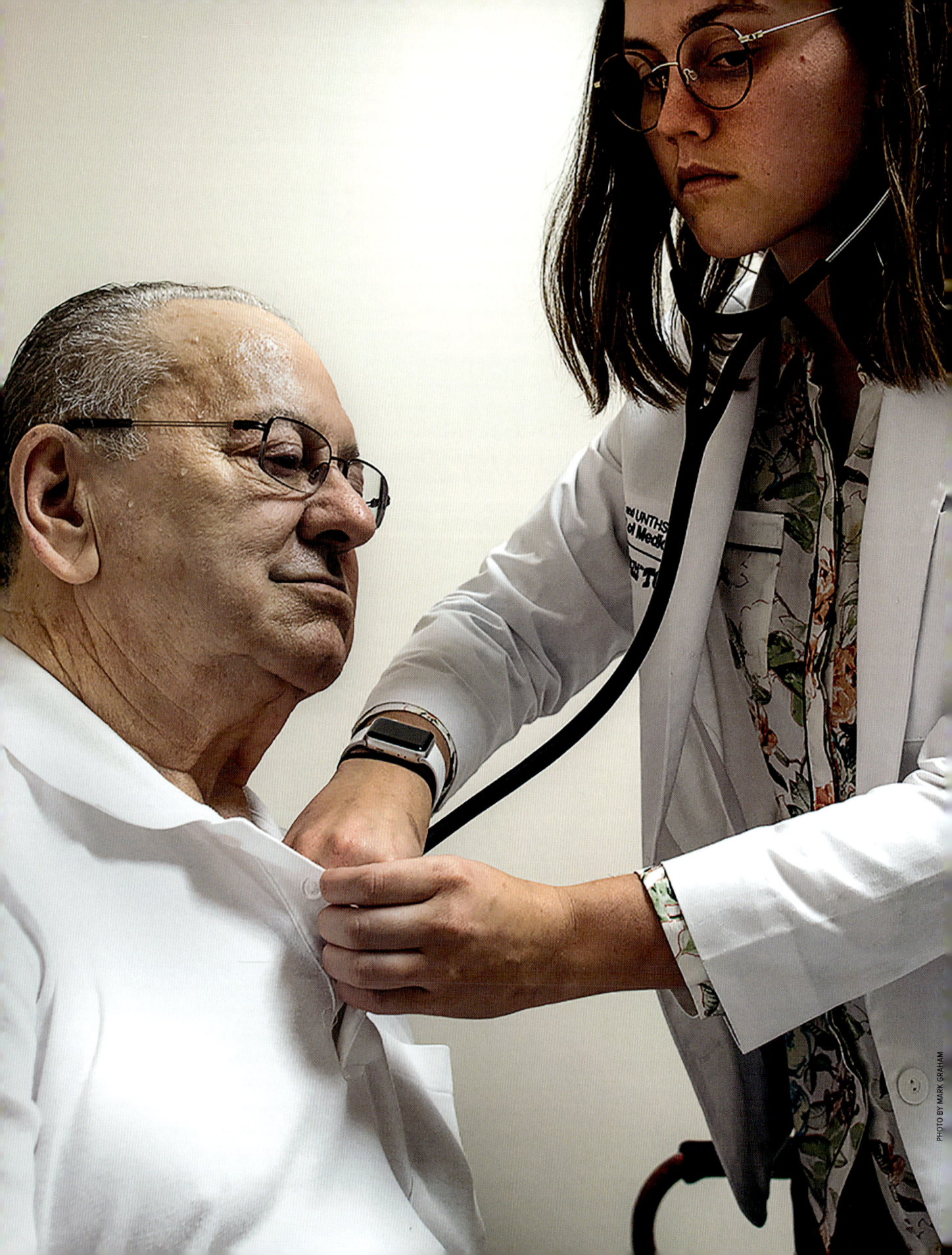

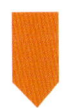

"If you've gone to a doctor and it doesn't feel like the conversation is formulaic, it means the doctor is good at what they are doing."

Jonas Kruse

* * *

Not every patient the TCU medical students interact with during their first year suffers real symptoms. They also work with professional actors like Melinda Massie, one of 90 women and men hired to perform as standardized patients.

In advance of every student encounter, Massie and her fellow standardized patients for that week's class attend a three- or four-hour training session where each receives a dossier on a case. Details of the individuals they are to portray include name; age; family life; medical, personal and family histories; education; diet; number of sexual partners; medicines and allergies. The actors also learn about the disease, disorder or condition that made their characters seek medical attention.

"We get down to extremely specific details like 'I have two golden labs named Duke and Paisley,' " Massie said. "And we are told about our personalities, if we are shy or outgoing, and how this particular patient would react to the student's questions."

The goal is for each student to have as close to the same experience as possible when they interview and examine their standardized patient. Cameras are mounted in exam rooms so realistic they even smell like a typical doctor's office. Members of the faculty watch the student-patient interactions from a control room.

Before stepping into the room, each student receives a folder with a patient's chief complaint and a nugget of information about the individual. During the patient exams, students are expected to ask questions in an organic way rather than sounding as if they are reading from a checklist or script. Afterward, they review video of the encounter and receive feedback from faculty, staff and the actor.

Esparza was performing a routine cardiac exam on a standardized patient when he detected something through his stethoscope that didn't sound right. Two doctors came and listened to the man's chest, agreeing they picked up a faint murmur. "It was a little scary," Esparza said.

"If you've gone to a doctor and it doesn't feel like the conversation is formulaic, it means the doctor is good at what they are doing," Kruse said. "It's not easy. I find that if a patient is more short with their answers, it gives me less time to formulate my next questions."

Losefsky walked out of her first graded encounter only to realize that she had neglected to ask about suicidal thoughts. "I figure it's better to forget now," she said, "than on a real patient."

Following the transition to telemedicine in the spring — a step many physicians around the country made out of necessity — Massie missed the energy of being around the students. She said she had to up her game when looking for their nonverbal cues to critique. For example, Massie might tell a student that "they scrunched up their eyebrows" when she said, while in character, that she had an open marriage. "Something like that might make a patient feel judged."

* * *

As health care workers around the country risked their lives in the fight against Covid-19, Losefsky, Kinard and their classmates said they had no qualms about their chosen profession.

Kruse, who was born in Germany and moved to the U.S. at age 3, spent many childhood hours in the hospital with his father, a geriatrician in San Clemente, California. Even before his class's springtime unit on neurology, Kruse gravitated to a future in acute neurological care, treating strokes, seizures and more.

Inspired by her immigrant mother, a one-time janitor and restaurant cook, Avila entered medical school with the goal of working with women. Her mom had never had a women's health care provider with whom she could communicate in her native tongue.

"I want Spanish-speaking women to feel empowered to speak for themselves about their sexual health and reproductive options with another woman who understands both their language and culture," Avila said.

Esparza said the pandemic gave him more time to ponder his four-year research project. Unlike the majority of U.S. medical schools, TCU requires students to pursue a single line of research leading up to a degree.

He studied the potential positive effects of exercise and neoadjuvant therapy — chemotherapy administered prior to surgery — on patients with gastrointestinal cancer. He looked at muscle strength, quality of life and other variables among patients who had completed chemotherapy to evaluate the role exercise and the additional therapy played in helping patients rebound faster following treatment.

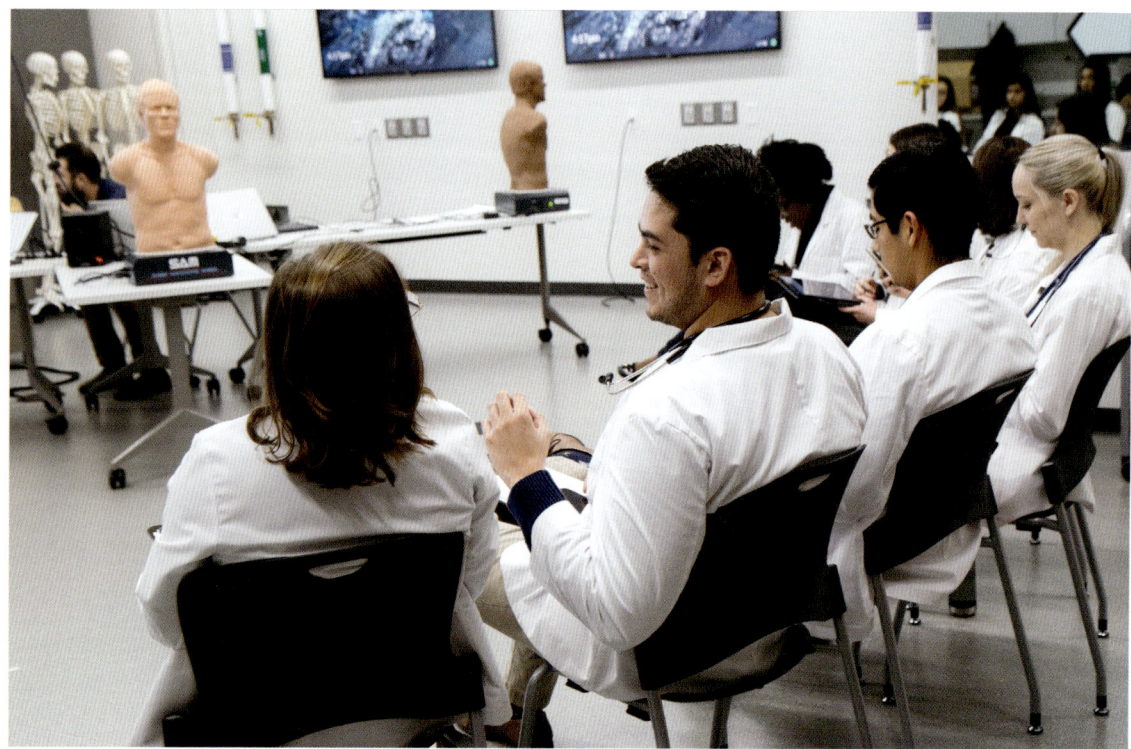

Above: Esparza joined classmates in a simulation classroom. Right: Kinard practiced her clinical skills.

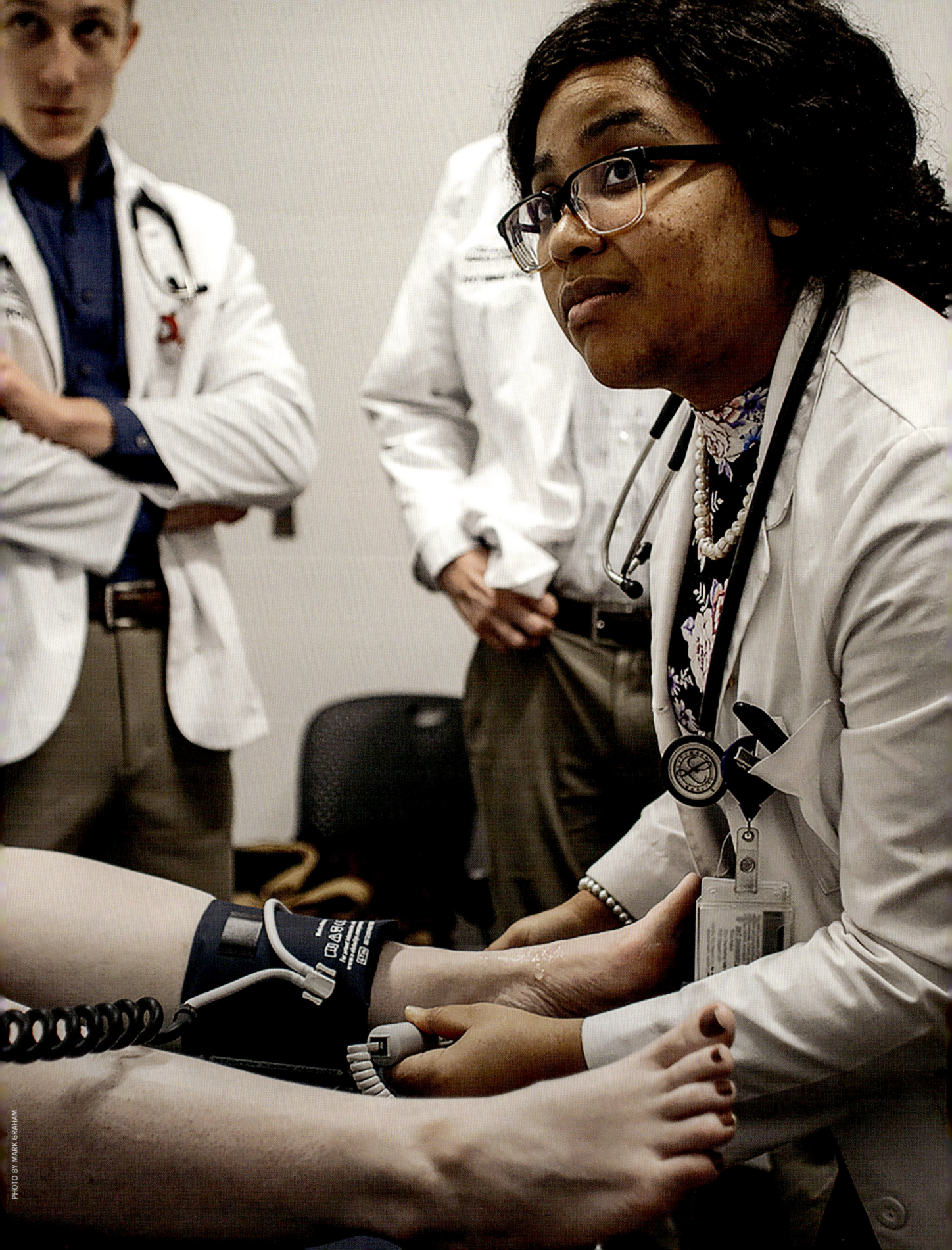

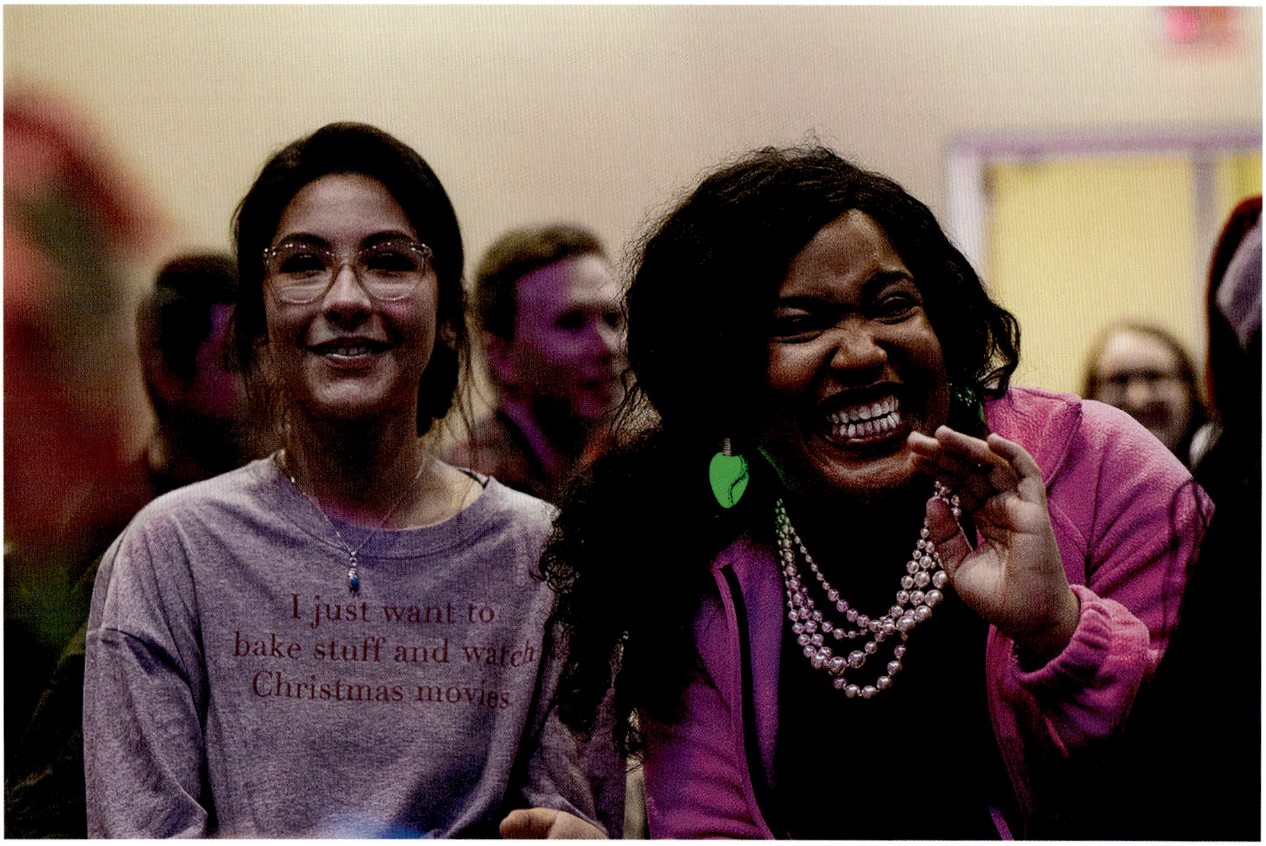

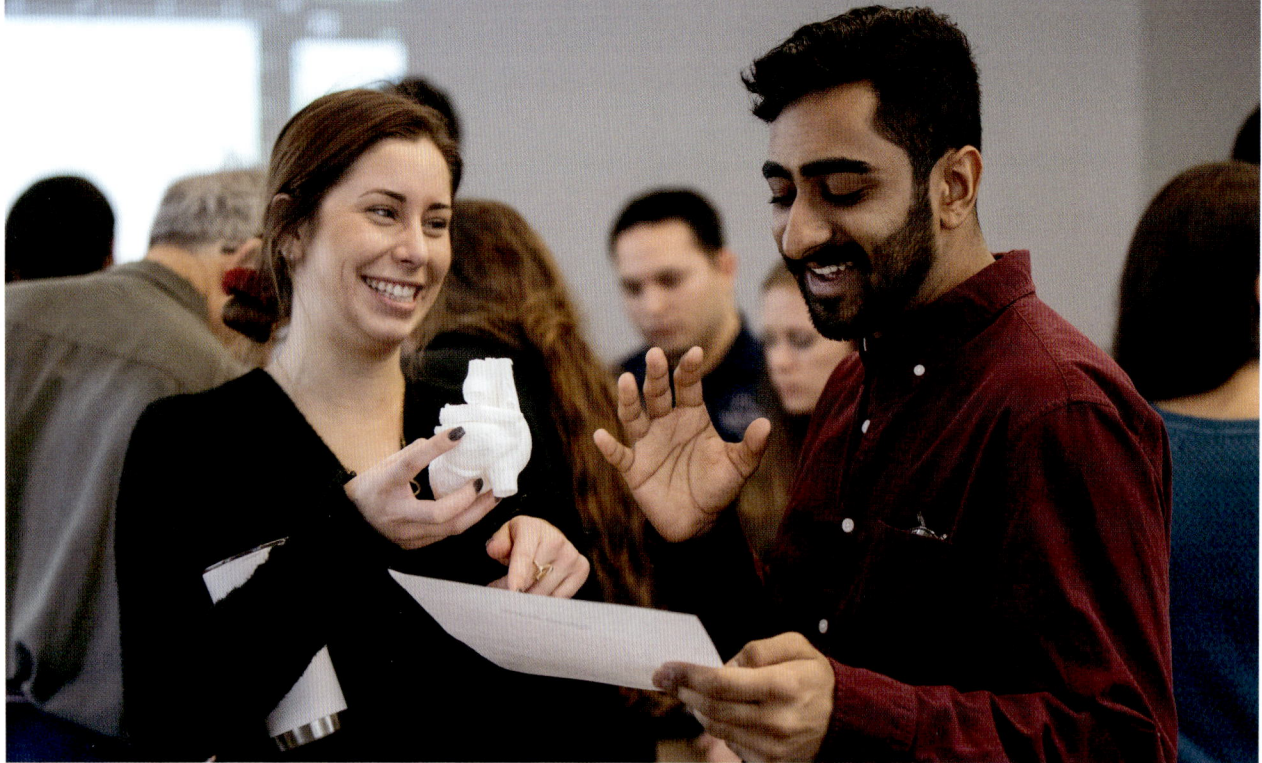

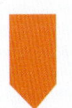

> "I want Spanish-speaking women to feel empowered to speak for themselves about their sexual health and reproductive options with another woman who understands both their language and culture."

Ive Avila

Top: Avila and Kinard enjoyed Winterfest 2019, which included a student talent show, baking contest and gift exchange.

Bottom: McKenna Chalman and Shah worked through instructions in a communication skills workshop.

* * *

Esparza and his classmates grappled with the pandemic's implications for health care professionals as the pandemic widened. Coronavirus deaths among health care workers, many of whom faced shortages of personal protective equipment early on, sent shockwaves through society.

The students found an ally in Flynn, who had been a young physician in the San Francisco area in the 1980s at the start of the AIDS crisis, when no one knew what caused the disease or how it spread. The dean was candid with the students about the fear and unease back then among members of the medical community. From the earliest days of the pandemic, he was also adamant about prioritizing student safety, a big factor in the school pausing clinical rotations.

Losefsky's response included holding herself to the highest ethical standards. She followed every guideline that came from the Centers for Disease Control and Prevention, which meant rigorous social distancing. She also answered a call in May 2020 for a blood drive. Losefsky's O negative blood type makes her a universal donor.

"Many of my classmates have organized various outreach efforts," she said. "I can donate my bodily fluids."

Shah supported a student-led effort to collect protective equipment for local physicians running low on or out of masks, gloves and other essentials. Kinard, Avila and classmate Kavneet Kaur collaborated on an effort to assist Samaritan House in Fort Worth, which provides permanent housing and support for 60 residents living with HIV and AIDS.

Kinard also harnessed social media to connect with physicians across the country. She created an account on Twitter, now X, to follow health care professionals and patients posting on the platform during isolation.

"It's interesting to absorb the information and acknowledge the missteps," she said, "so I'll be prepared in three years not to make the same mistakes."

Kruse devoted 72 hours to answering phones at Tarrant County's Covid-19 hotline. During a six-hour shift in March 2020, he fielded more than two dozen calls. Kruse talked the callers through whether they should go to the hospital, seek out a test for the virus — which was hard to find at that point — or stay at home.

"As first-year medical students, we're not really an asset in terms of workflow right now, but we've gotten a lot more clinical experiences than most other first-years," said Kruse, who volunteered to trace coronavirus contacts by phone that May. "It doesn't feel good to do nothing."

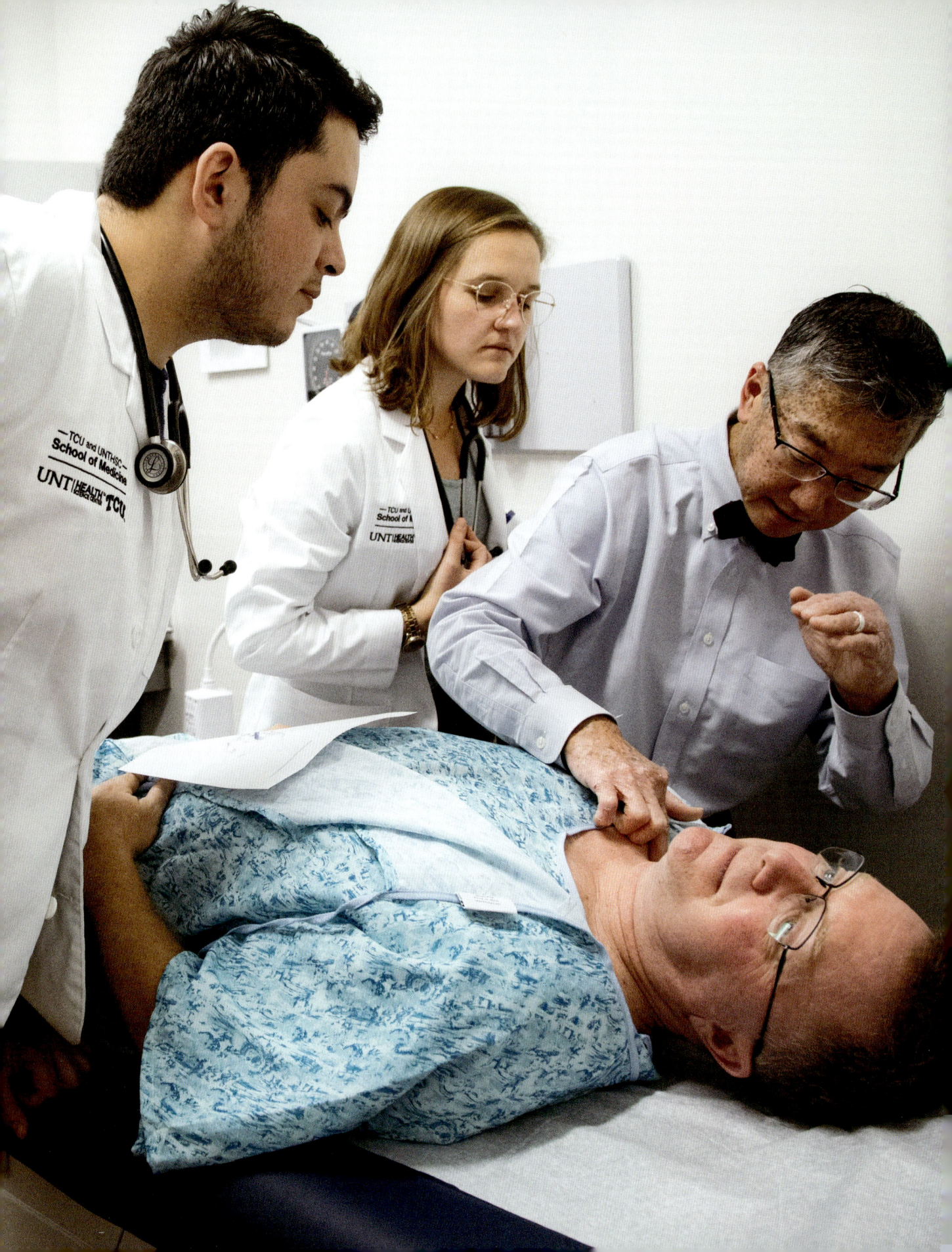

As the students wrapped up the initial year of medical school, they had acquired a baseline in clinical sciences, including a foundational understanding of major organs and body systems. They'd learned about anatomy, mental illness and life cycles using everything from high-tech simulations to handwritten flashcards. They knew their way around a stethoscope, a skill that takes years to master.

"They also understand disease and death about 10 years earlier than their peers," said Flynn, echoing something he'd been told during his own days as a medical student at the University of Michigan. "Very quickly you realize this is not a TV show. You develop both a respect and fear for diseases and death."

Looking back on a year that defied expectations, the students seemed united in their excitement for the future. "This past year went so much faster than I expected," Losefsky said. "But whenever I missed the group, I'd remind myself that these people are going to be my colleagues forever."

The year also flew by for Kruse, who in April 2020 bought a house in Fort Worth with his wife. He'd met Anabel while they were undergraduates at Baylor University.

During the white coat ceremony at the start of the academic year, Kruse drew laughs when he remarked that he and his fellow students "were about to become physicians in a short seven to 10 years."

In the intervening months, a gravitas had settled on him, particularly given the speed of his first year of medical school, along with its twists and turns.

"I keep telling myself that if I can do this, I can do the next level," he said.

"One step at a time."

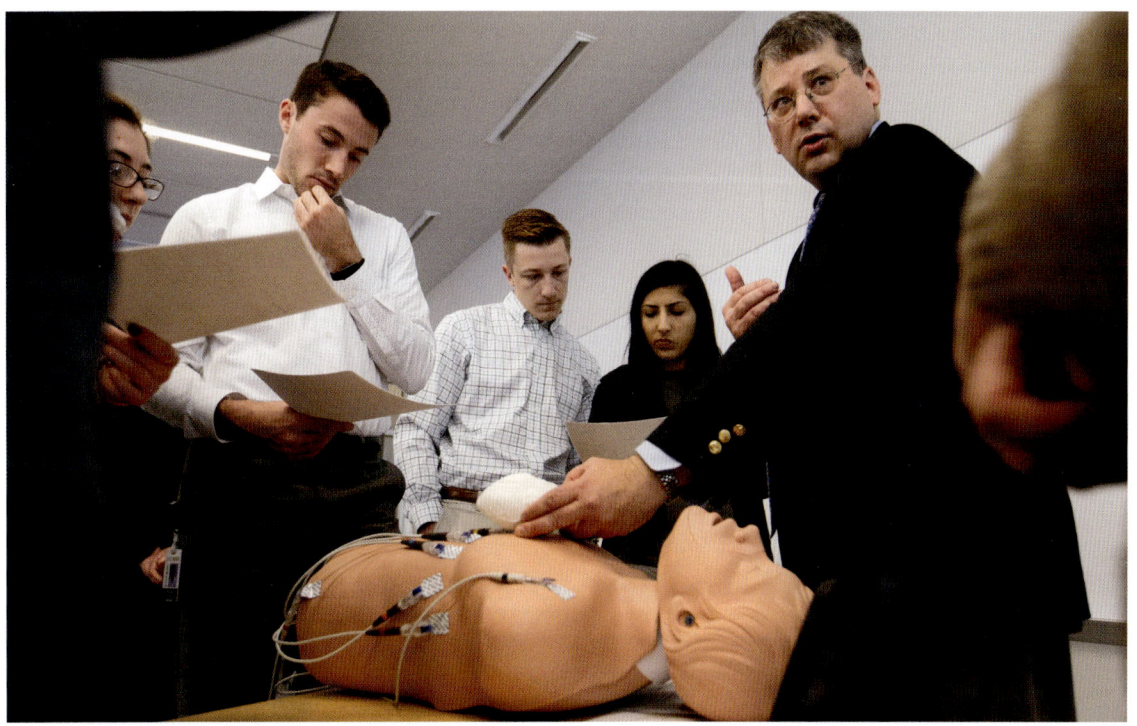

Above: Flanked by Helena Kons, Tom Roser and Sarah Cheema, Kruse, center, listened to instruction by professor Kevin Kunkler.
Left: Esparza and Shelby Wildish observed Dr. Song Lee with standardized patient Chris Clark.

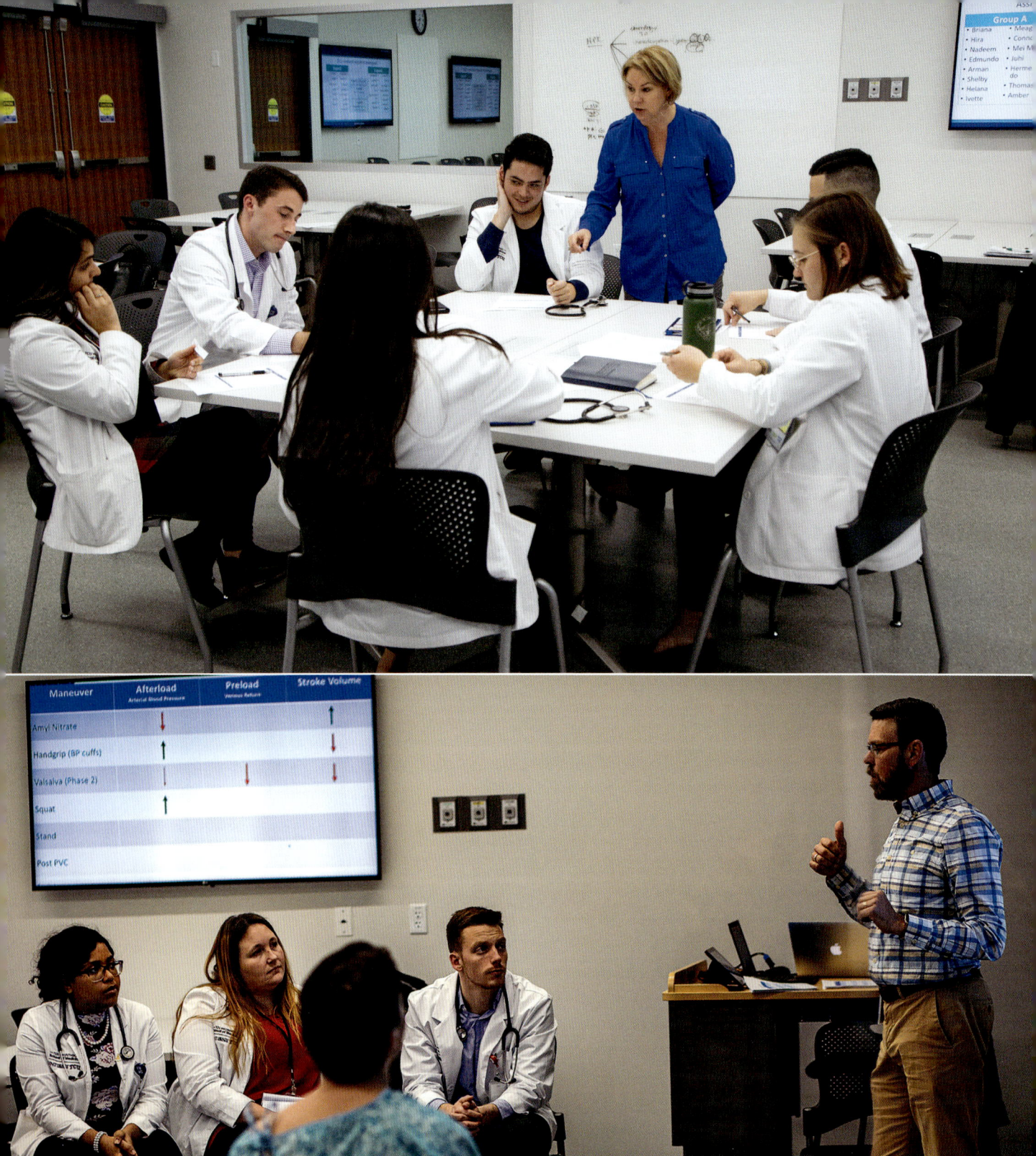

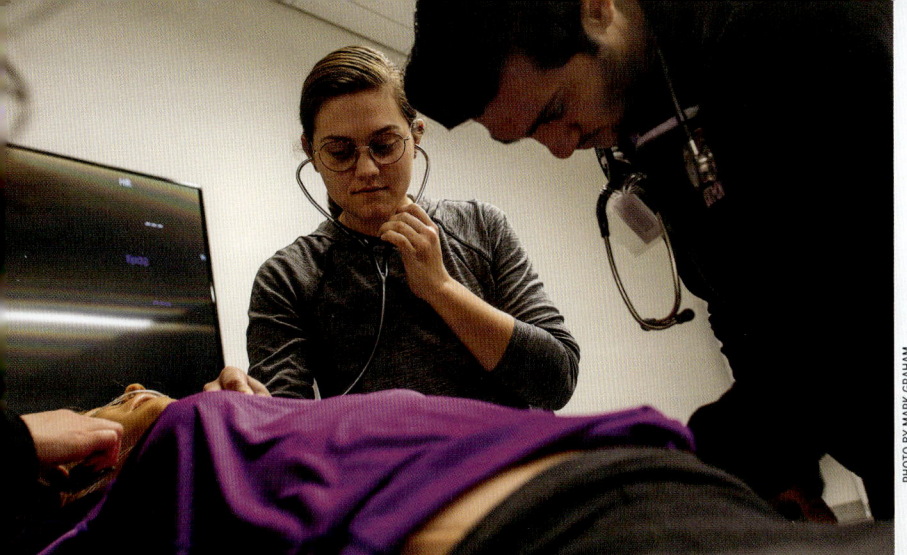

PHOTO BY MARK GRAHAM

Opposite page, top:

Esparza and fellow students worked with the medical school's founding artistic director, Valeri Lantz-Gefroh, on a role-playing exercise to enhance communication skills.

Dr. James Furgerson led a class that included Kinard, Stephanie Schaumberg and Glen Smith in advance of students' clinical skills sessions.

This page, from top:

Losefsky and fellow first-year medical student Nadeem Al-Adli practiced on a manikin during a pulmonary lab session.

Phil Hartman, emeritus dean and professor of biology in TCU's College of Science & Engineering, left, consulted with Dr. Mohanakrishnan Sathyamoorthy, chair of internal medicine at the Burnett School of Medicine, and area businessman Sathishkumar Gopalaswamy while judging student presentations.

Kruse examined standardized patient Michael Carver-Simmons in the clinical skills lab.

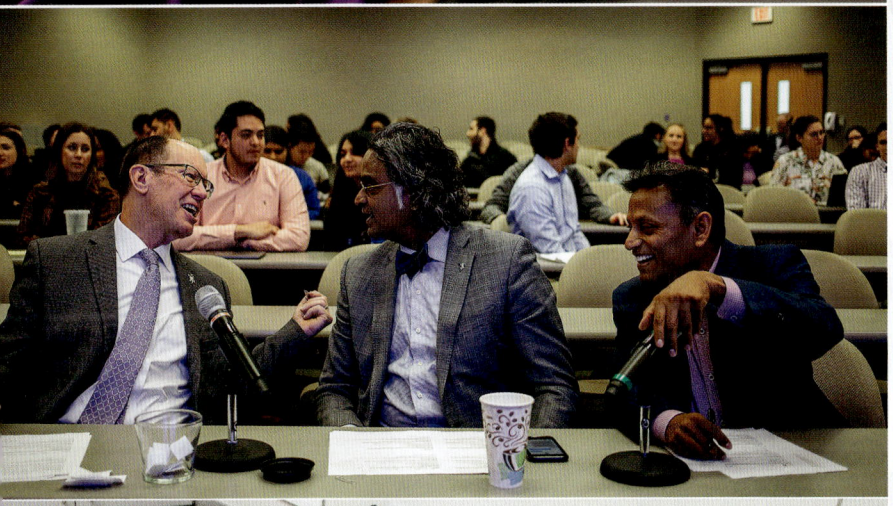

PHOTO BY MARK GRAHAM

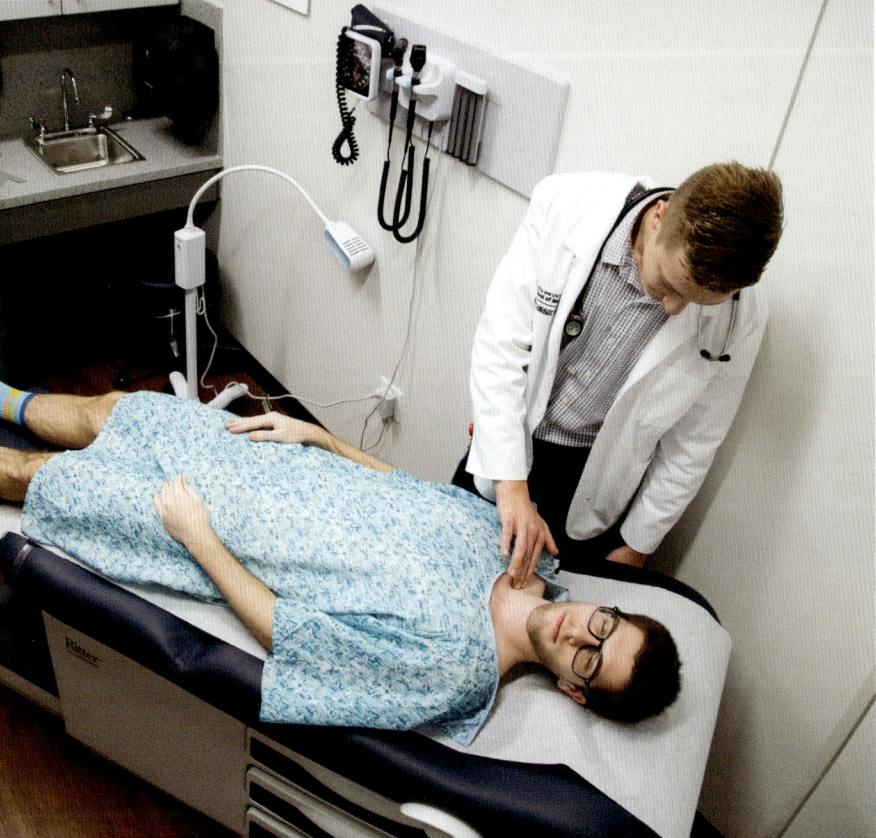

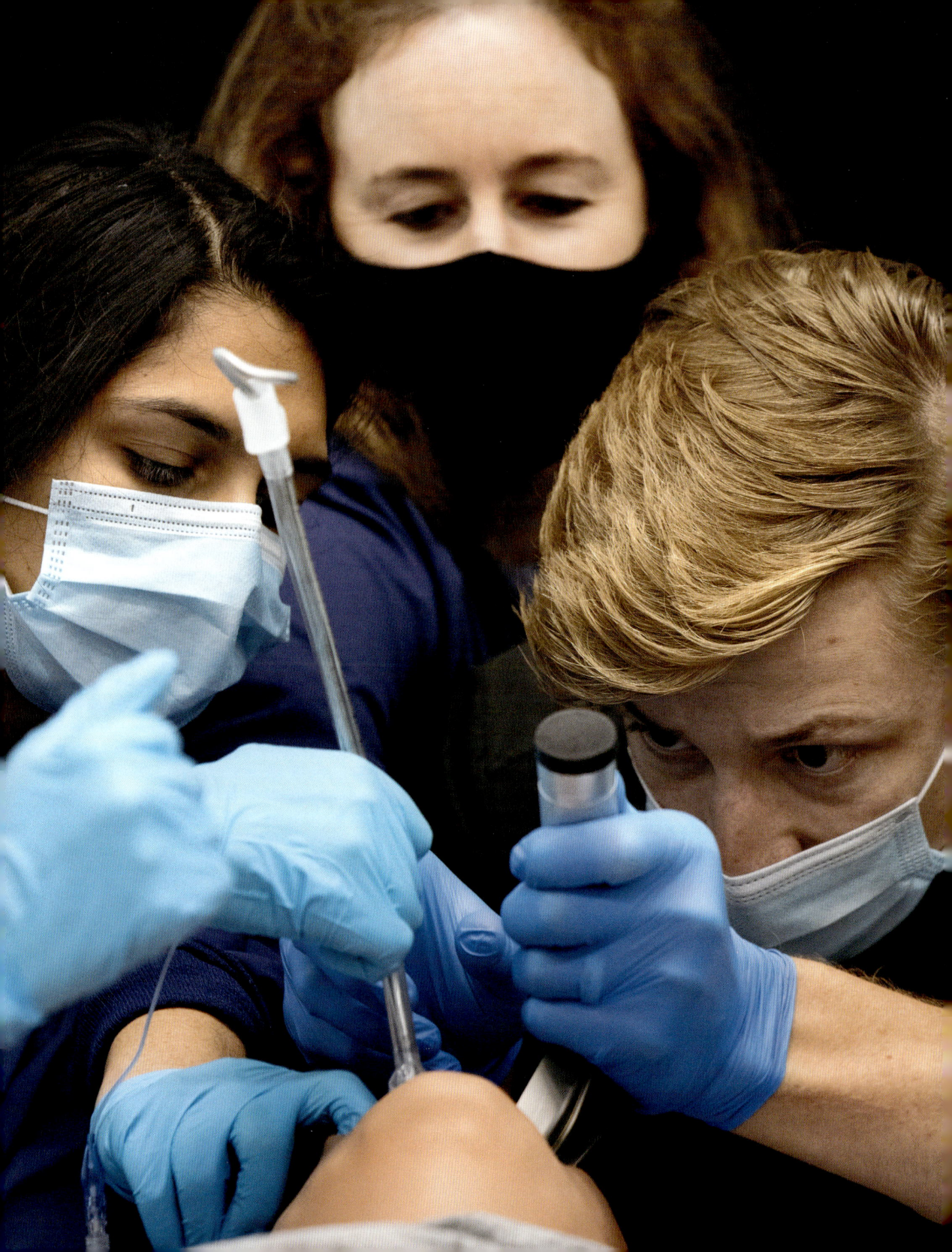

YEAR TWO

2020-21

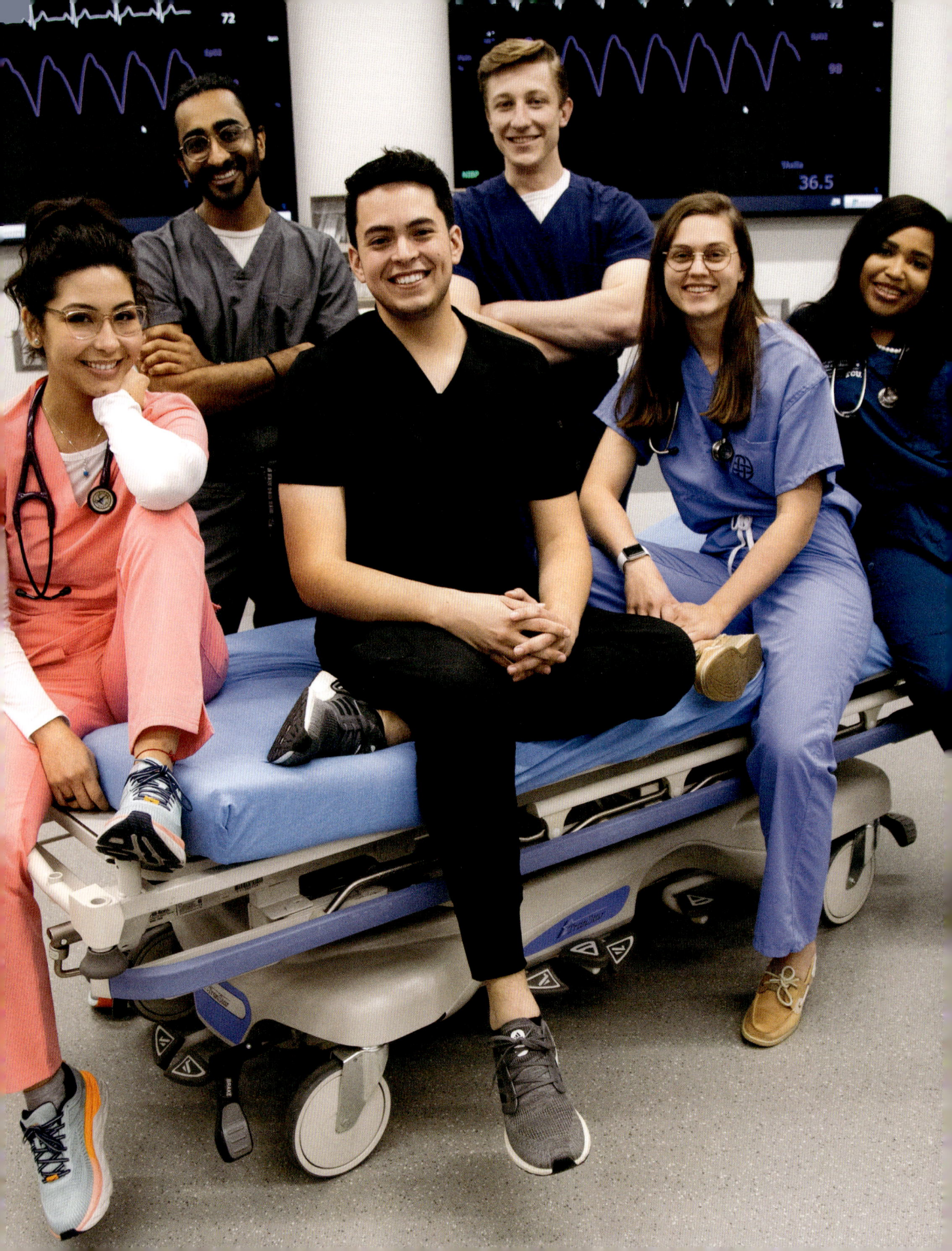

Empathetic Scholars

The second year of medical school for the Class of 2023 coincided with a time of deep division in the nation. On the first Tuesday in November 2020, Joe Biden defeated incumbent Donald Trump to become president of the United States in a highly contentious race with wide-ranging consequences.

America's opioid crisis had surged during the pandemic. Nearly 69,000 deaths were attributed to the extremely addictive class of drugs, representing a 44 percent increase over the previous year and more than triple the total from a decade earlier.

Covid-19 caused profound societal fissures as many Americans rebelled against mask mandates and social distancing. Another point of controversy arose when schools around the country delayed a return to in-person instruction in fall 2020, with many opting for online-only or hybrid schedules.

By the end of 2020, the CDC reported that Covid-19 had killed 350,000 Americans, with more than 20 million confirmed cases.

In December 2020, the first Covid vaccines were administered in the U.S. Mass immunization efforts gained speed in the new year. By March 2021, 100 million vaccine doses had been given to Americans; two-thirds of the population had received at least one shot by June of that year.

The public health crisis drew attention to another problem brewing: The Association of American Medical Colleges estimated that by the year 2034, the United States could see shortfalls of up to 124,000 doctors nationwide.

* * *

The Class of 2023's second year of medical school, which began in July 2020, focused on mentorship and training in the field rather than the classroom. The 58 returning students worked all year in area hospitals alongside doctors, nurses, physician assistants and other health care professionals. They learned while observing and doing.

Unlike most medical students in the U.S., TCU's students enter Year 2 with significant clinical experience. At that point, they've also received extensive training in empathy, compassion and interpersonal skills.

"It's a very rare opportunity to create a medical school from scratch," Judy Bernas, senior associate dean, said of a curriculum designed to prepare students to become better doctors, colleagues and leaders. "When six of us were sitting around a table long before the first students stepped on campus, we found ourselves talking a lot about empathy and communication.

"We began focusing on creating Empathetic Scholars®, which really captured what we wanted to do here," she said. "What we all learned during the

Ive Avila, Dilan Shah, Edmundo Esparza, Jonas Kruse, Quinn Losefsky and Charna Kinard faced an unexpected global pandemic early in their medical education, but the crisis only strengthened their resolve to serve humanity through careers in medicine.

pandemic was that empathy became very important not just for our patients but for our caregivers, to take care of each other and how they treated themselves."

Erin Nelson, assistant dean of physician communication, had been a colleague of Bernas and Dean Stuart D. Flynn at the University of Arizona College of Medicine–Phoenix before they recruited her to TCU in 2017. She said the Burnett School of Medicine seeks to enroll future doctors who are driven by connection, community and contribution.

"We know that even if someone is brilliant, if they aren't as interested in interaction with team-based care or team-based learning, they won't be a good fit for our school," Nelson said. "We are trying to change the landscape of both how students are trained and how they will set out on a lifelong manner of engaging with their patients, their patients' families and their community."

* * *

From the earliest days of their hospital rotations, a gravitas settled on Dilan Shah, Quinn Losefsky, Emundo Esparza, Charna Kinard, Jonas Kruse and Ive Avila.

Early in his second year, Shah put his Empathetic Scholar® training to use with the family of a patient he'd known since his first month of medical school. He had seen the woman regularly as part of his family medicine clerkship, the only rotation starting in Year 1. During his surgery rotation, Shah participated in all three of the patient's surgeries for diverticulitis, an infection in the intestines. When the surgeon opened the patient up a final time, he and Shah were shocked to find that the small bowel had died. They immediately stitched up the woman's abdomen and went to break the dire news to her family.

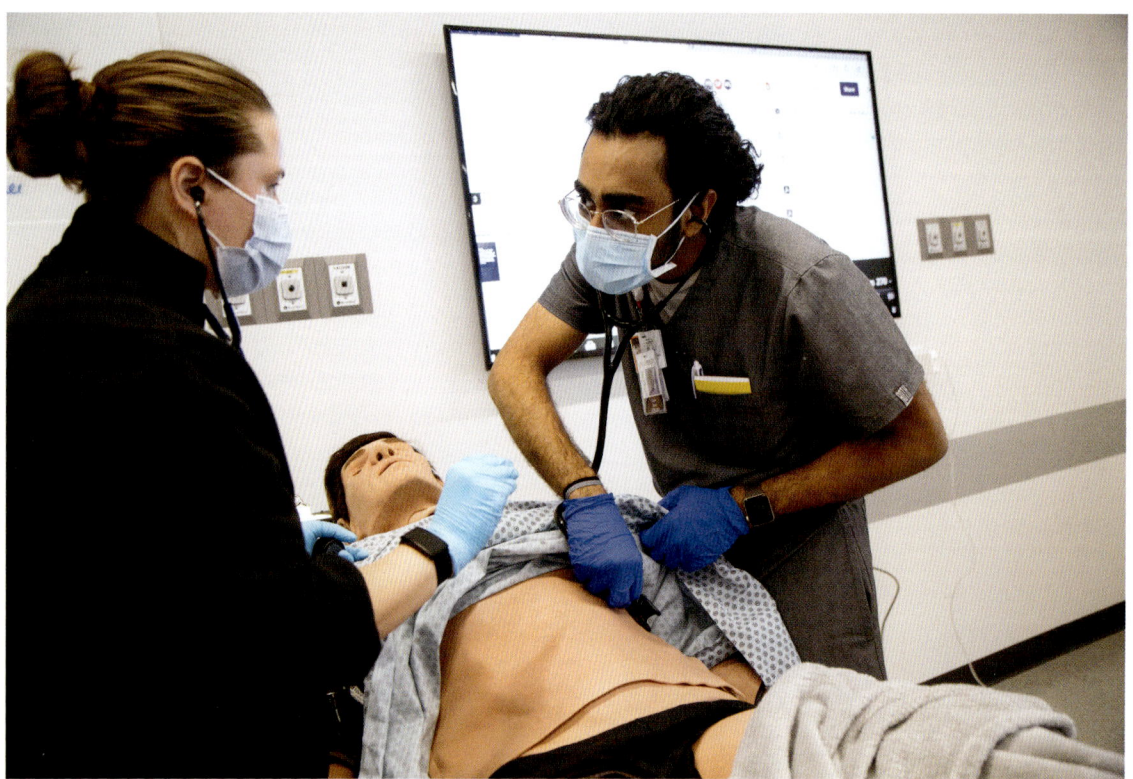

Above: Sam Evans and Shah examined a manikin to diagnose lung diseases. Right: Shah was elected president of the medical school's student senate during Year 2.

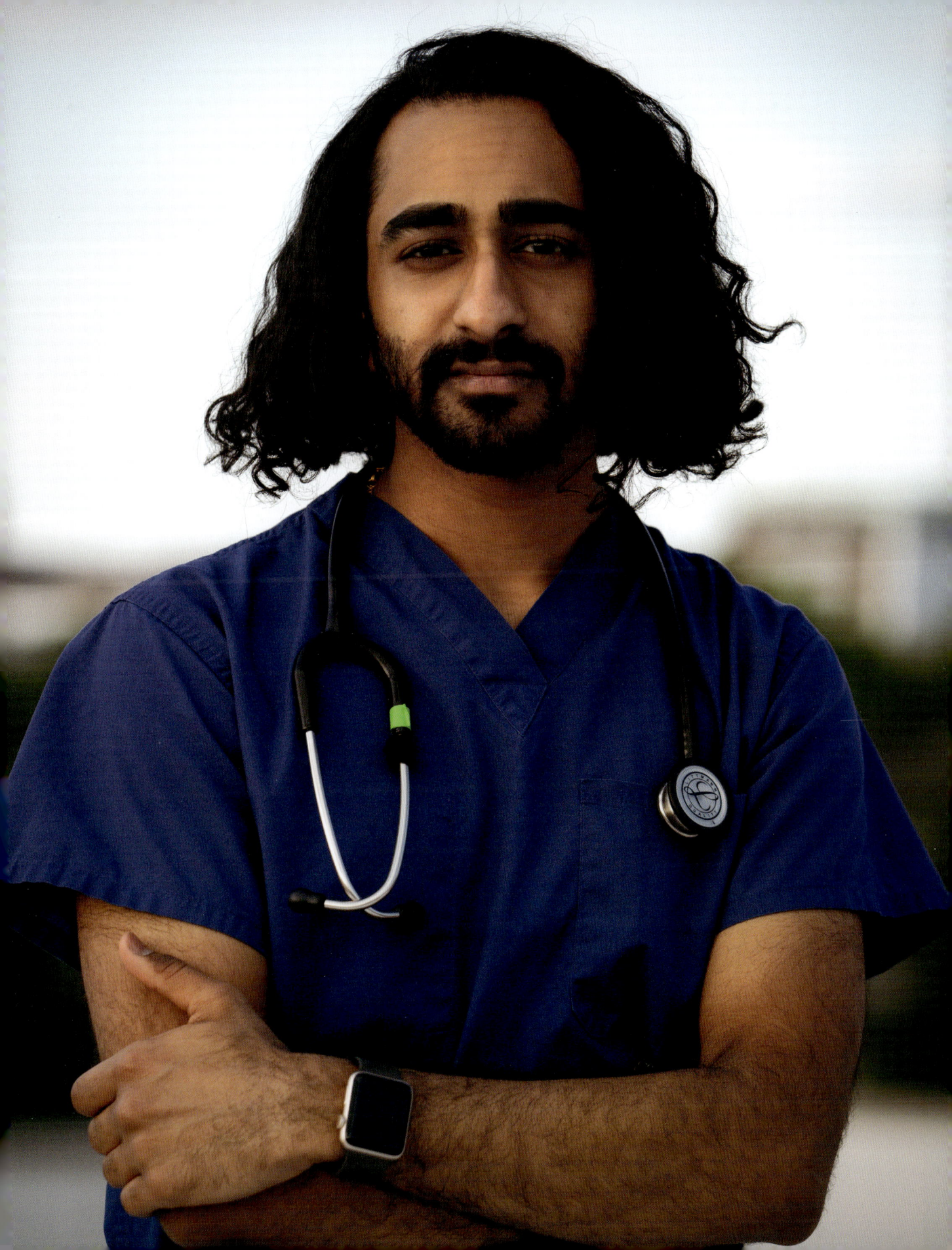

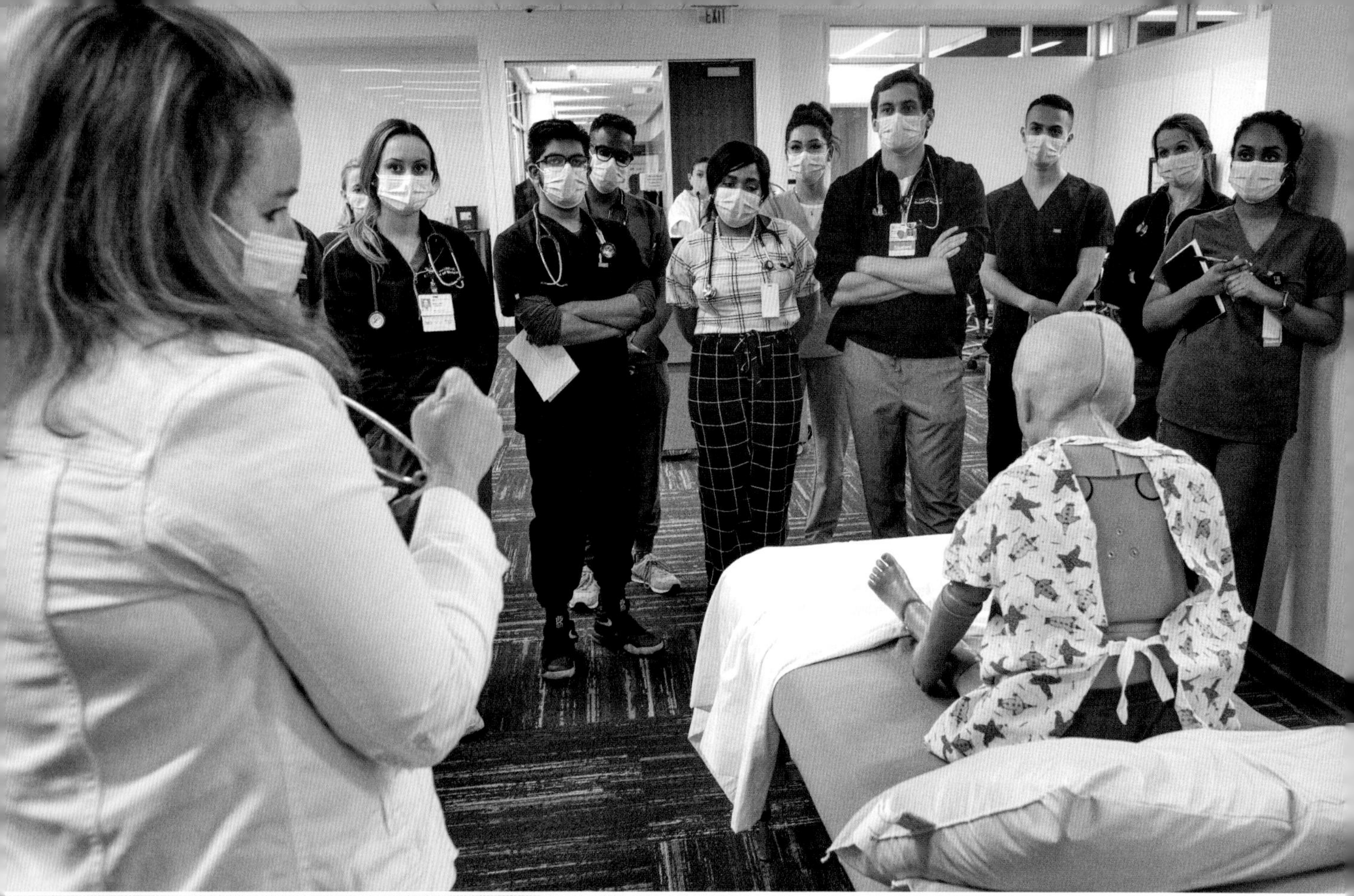
EXIT

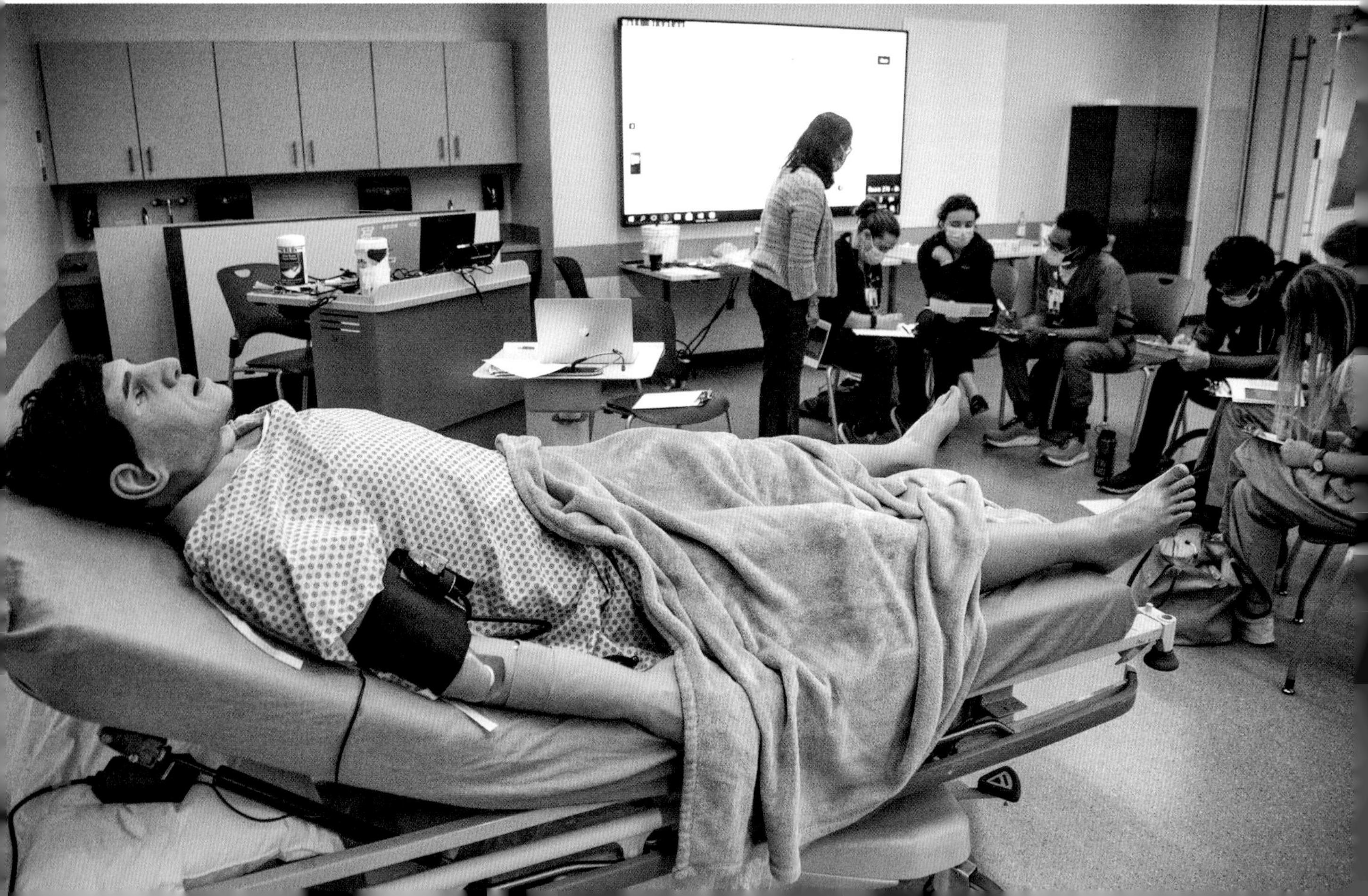

Top: Dr. Hannah Smitherman, an emergency room physician, led a class for second-year medical students.

Bottom: Clinical skills are a huge emphasis in the second year of medical school at TCU.

Covid-19 restrictions meant only one family member was allowed in the waiting room, in this case the patient's daughter. Because she'd accompanied her mother on visits to the clinic, Shah knew her too. After the surgeon left, Shah offered to escort the daughter downstairs to meet with other family members. Through her sobs, she asked if he would share the prognosis with them.

"When you go over bad news, you have to be way more repetitive and intentional, and you have to be slow and kind," Shah said. "You need to pay attention to how the patient's family is feeling." The experience made him even more grateful to attend a medical school that emphasizes communication skills, he said.

The woman died on his last day of the rotation. Shah, whose interests that second year shifted from psychiatry to otolaryngology — a specialty that ranges from head and neck surgery to treatment of the ear, nose and throat — stayed in touch with her daughter.

"I am an eager student of medicine, but at the same time it's sad," Shah said. "This stuff gets really heavy."

Avila recalled a harrowing first week working in her future specialty. "I went from delivering a mother's worst nightmare in one room to another's dream come true with a perfect delivery in the next room.

"The happy mother loses sleep with her crying baby, and the baby-less mother wishes her baby's crying kept her awake," Avila said. "This week I learned the definition of medicine. It means holding her hand, being a friend, being an anything-she-needs."

Because the pandemic prevented the Class of 2023 from meeting in person from mid-March until September 2020, faculty and administrators retooled the second-year curriculum to include five weeks of intensive classroom training before the students were dispatched to hospitals. They learned how to check someone into the hospital and intubate a patient during an emergency. They also performed pediatrics exams using replicas of babies.

Losefsky volunteered to go first to conduct an introductory exam on "Oliver," the 6- to 9-month-old electronic manikin. She looked at its eyes, heart and lungs before checking the pulse in the femoral artery with her fingertips.

"It's funny how much of medicine is subjective," Losefsky told Kruse after he took his turn. "You know it when you feel it."

Later that week, Kruse, Losefsky and Shah spent an afternoon suturing fake skin under the watchful eye of Shanna Combs, an OB-GYN who graduated from TCU in 2001 with a degree in ballet. YouTube videos of suturing techniques played on iPads directly in front of the students as they worked first with yarn, then nylon and different types of needles.

"When you have a uterine artery pulsating at you, your knot tying is all muscle memory," Combs told the students as they prepared for nine weeks of immersions in North Texas hospitals.

"Unless you grew up in the world of a hospital — some students have, but most have not — there's nothing that can compare to the first day you walk into this large hustling and bustling edifice, which takes your breath away," Flynn said.

From October to December 2020, the students spent three weeks focusing on internal medicine, a week in pediatrics, two weeks in OB-GYN and three weeks in surgery.

"The energy of the hospital is amazing," Esparza said. "You feel like you are part of something a lot larger than you are when you're there."

Kruse said he appreciated the additional training after doing a suture to sew up a cesarean section. When the attending physician praised Kruse's work, the new mother jokingly asked from the other side of the drape, "Is one of you teaching the other?"

Hospital shifts could stretch beyond the 12-hour mark. Most of the students brought textbooks with them to squeeze in extra studying in the doctors' lounge, but the amount of downtime they had depended on the day.

"At the hospital when I'm seeing patients and learning, it's all fires blazing and I have energy, but when I get home, it hits," Kinard said. "Do I feel like a doctor? No. But I do feel like an effective empathetic scholar. I tell every patient that although I don't have all of the medical knowledge to heal them yet, I am here to be their advocate and make sure they feel heard."

* * *

Covid-19 continued to loom over the second year of medical school for the Class of 2023.

Although the medical students weren't allowed to care for Covid patients or work in areas where anyone infected with the virus was treated, they nonetheless suited up in protective gear for every

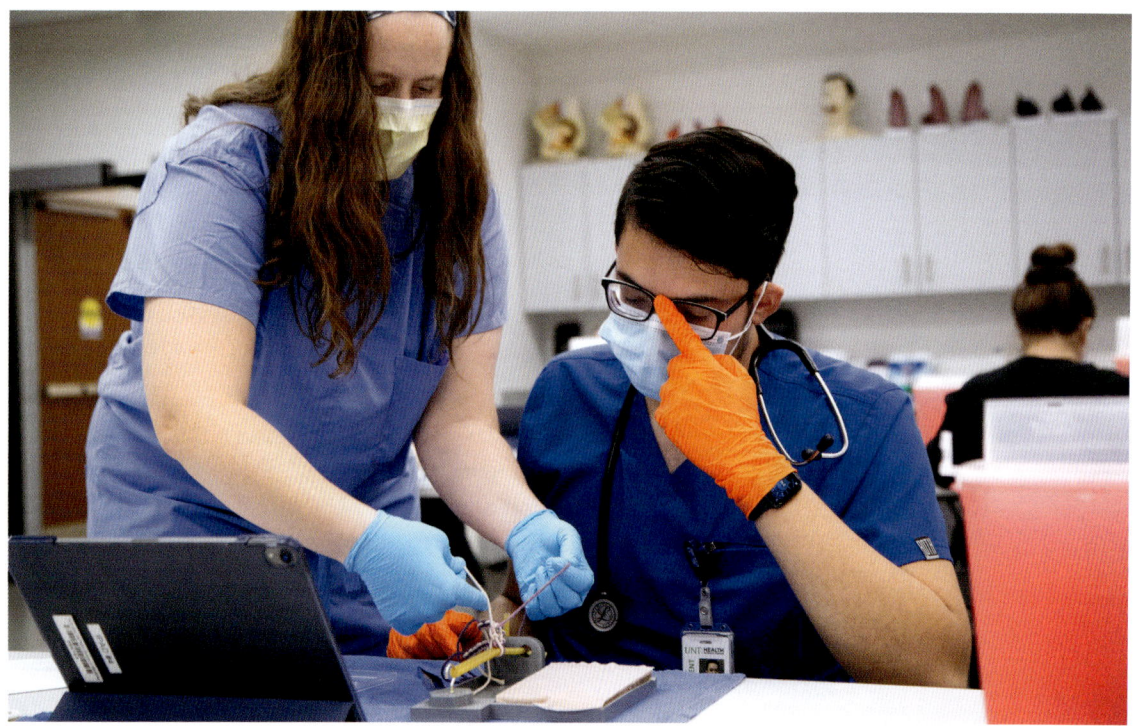

Above: Esparza learned suturing and knot tying alongside Dr. Shanna Combs, who majored in ballet as an undergraduate at TCU.
Right: Esparza sharpened his skills in advance of second-year surgical rotations at area hospitals.

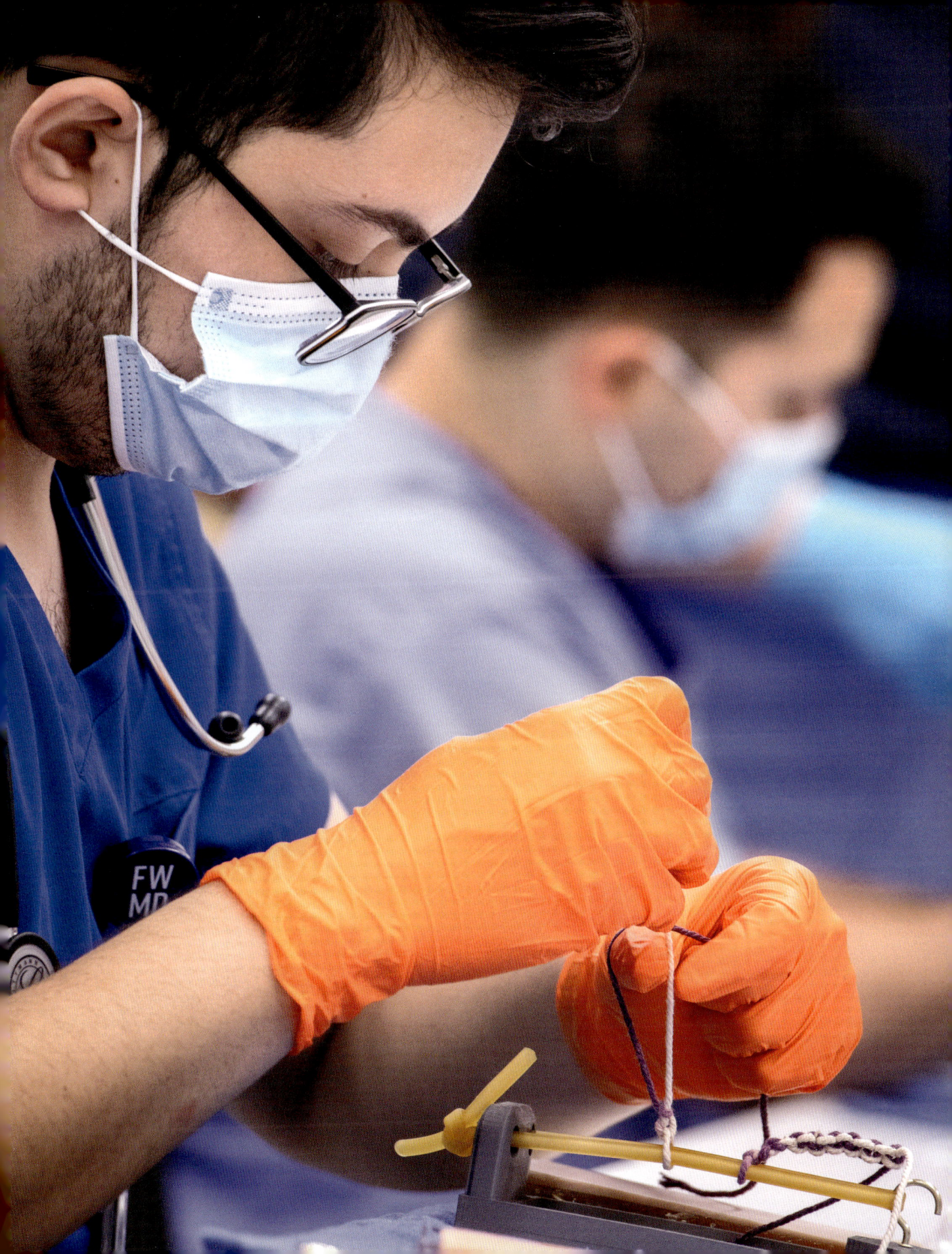

shift. Before their hospital rotations began, they attended a class to learn the proper way to scrub their hands and arms, tie surgical masks and make bouffant blue caps stay put.

"There are all these tricks to putting things on the right way to keep everything sterile," said Avila as she dressed in full surgical garb for the first time.

Kinard's strategy for keeping safe from the virus included staying in Fort Worth for Thanksgiving and Christmas 2020 rather than traveling to Chicago to see family.

Despite a negative Covid test before heading home for the holidays, Esparza worried that he might somehow infect his mother or siblings. "I've already lost one parent and need to protect the other," he said. "My anxiety was to the max over winter break."

A potential exposure in November 2020 forced Kruse to miss two weeks of surgical rotation, which he elected to make up over the winter holidays. Also as a precaution, Shah skipped the final week of his

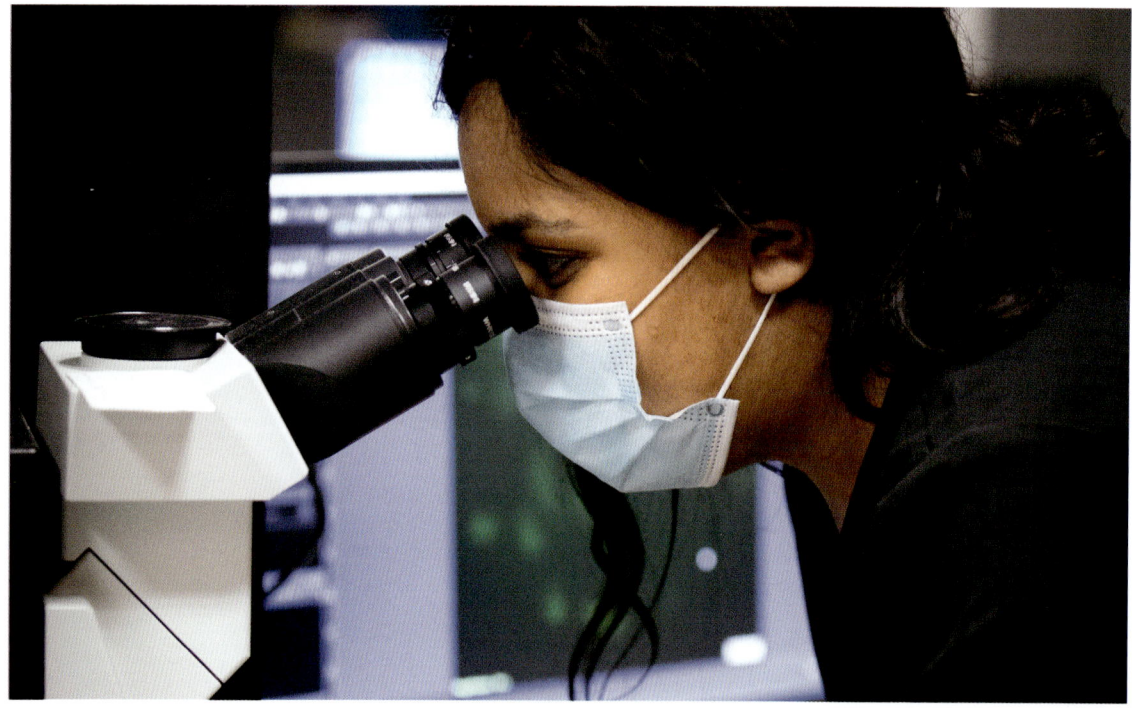

Above: For her senior thesis project, Kinard conducted research on nanotechnology in the lab of Anton Naumov, an associate professor of physics at TCU. Right: Kinard and fellow medical student Meaghan Rousset refined their techniques for examining a baby.

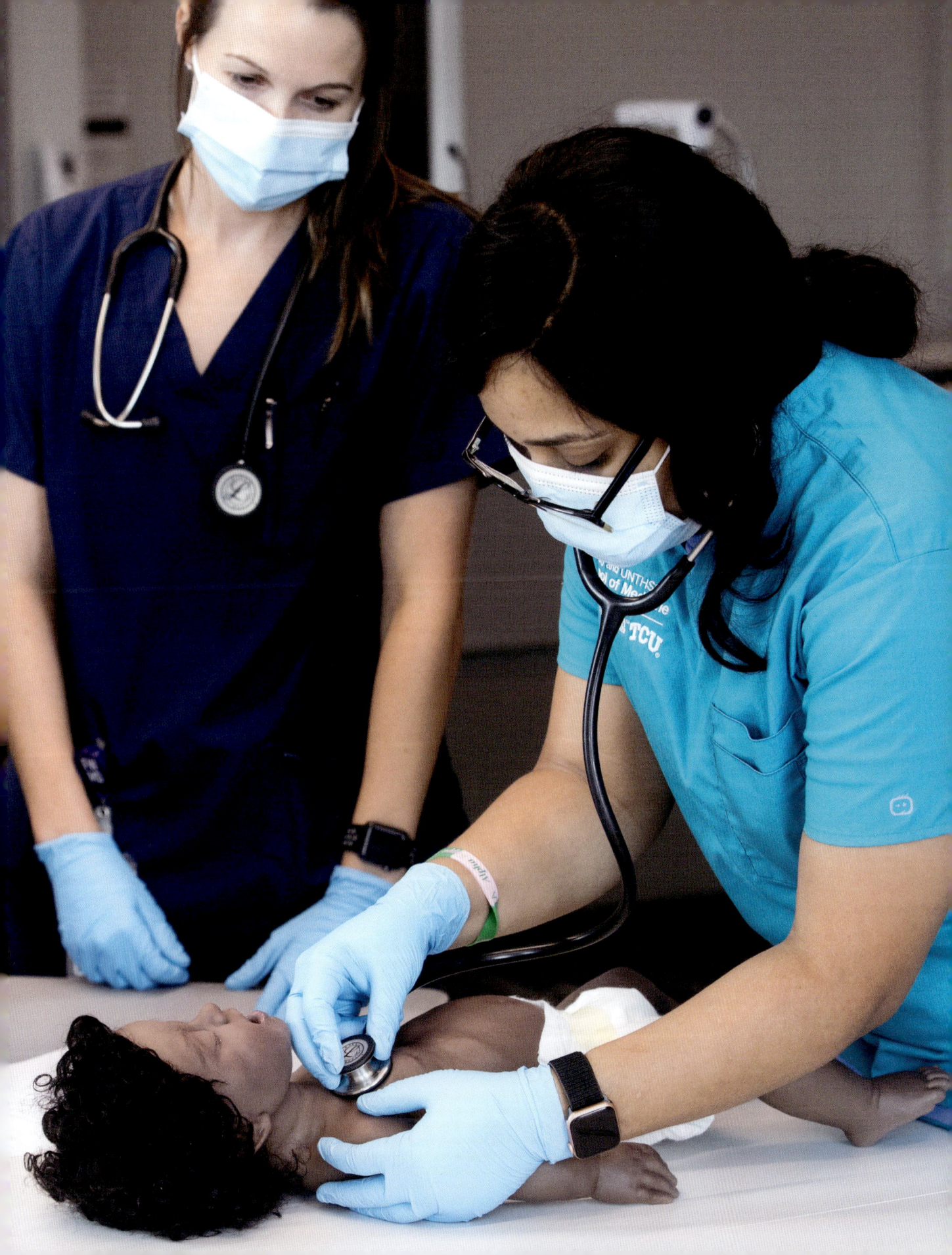

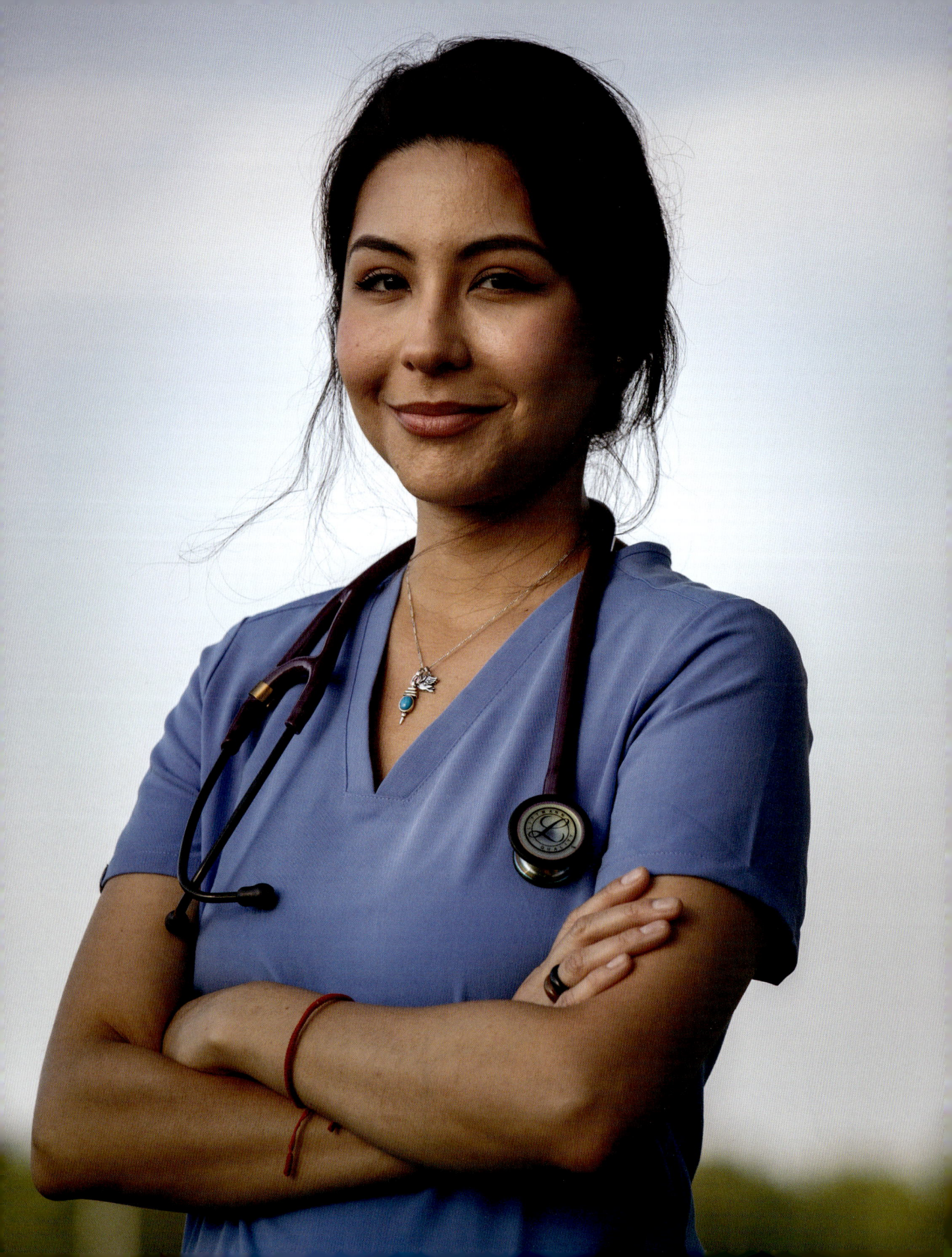

internal medicine rotation at a Dallas hospital. Neither fell ill.

Not so with Avila and her husband, who had bought a home a mile from the TCU main campus in fall 2020. They came down with Covid following the funeral of Sam's father. Both rebounded without any lingering effects but shared a respect for the contagious disease.

"It was pretty awful," Sam said.

"And could have been so much worse," said his wife, who missed the final week of her surgery rotation while ill.

Nearly all of the students received their first round of Covid vaccines at TCU days before the new year.

"We've been dealing with the pandemic since March, and everyone is fatigued," Kinard said.

"Getting the vaccine was about more than just protecting ourselves. It was about leading by example."

Losefsky interrupted her winter break to drive up for the day from Austin, Texas, to receive her first dose. "It was this huge weight off of my shoulders," she said. "I was actually surprised by how relieved I felt."

Shah met a handful of classmates at TCU's Brown-Lupton Health Center so they could get vaccinated together. He described the atmosphere as bordering on festive. "It was a great day for science."

* * *

In his role as the inaugural president of the medical school's student senate, Shah collaborated with several classmates to create a flyer aimed at explaining the vaccine to the public. "We're all

Left: Midway through medical school, Avila grew even more convinced about a career centered on delivering babies and working with women on reproductive health. Below: Dr. Karen Goff, a Fort Worth pediatrician, coached Avila as she checked the femoral artery pulse in an electronic baby intended to resemble a 6- to 9-month-old.

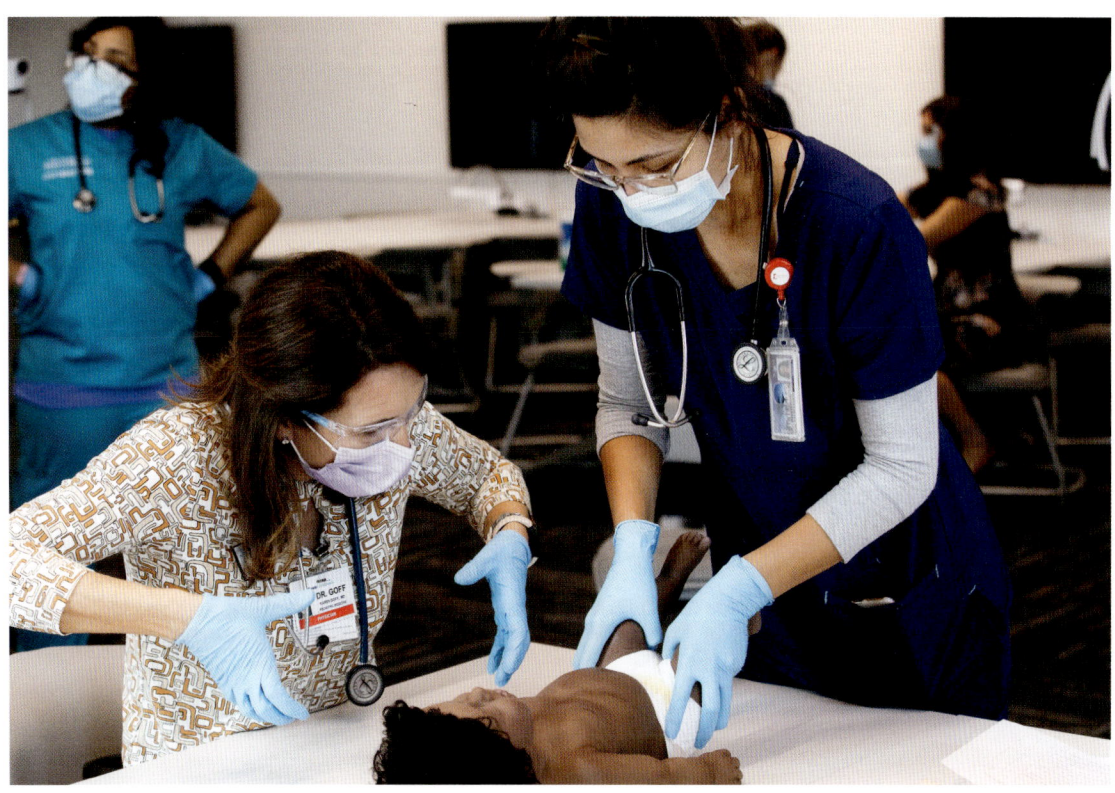

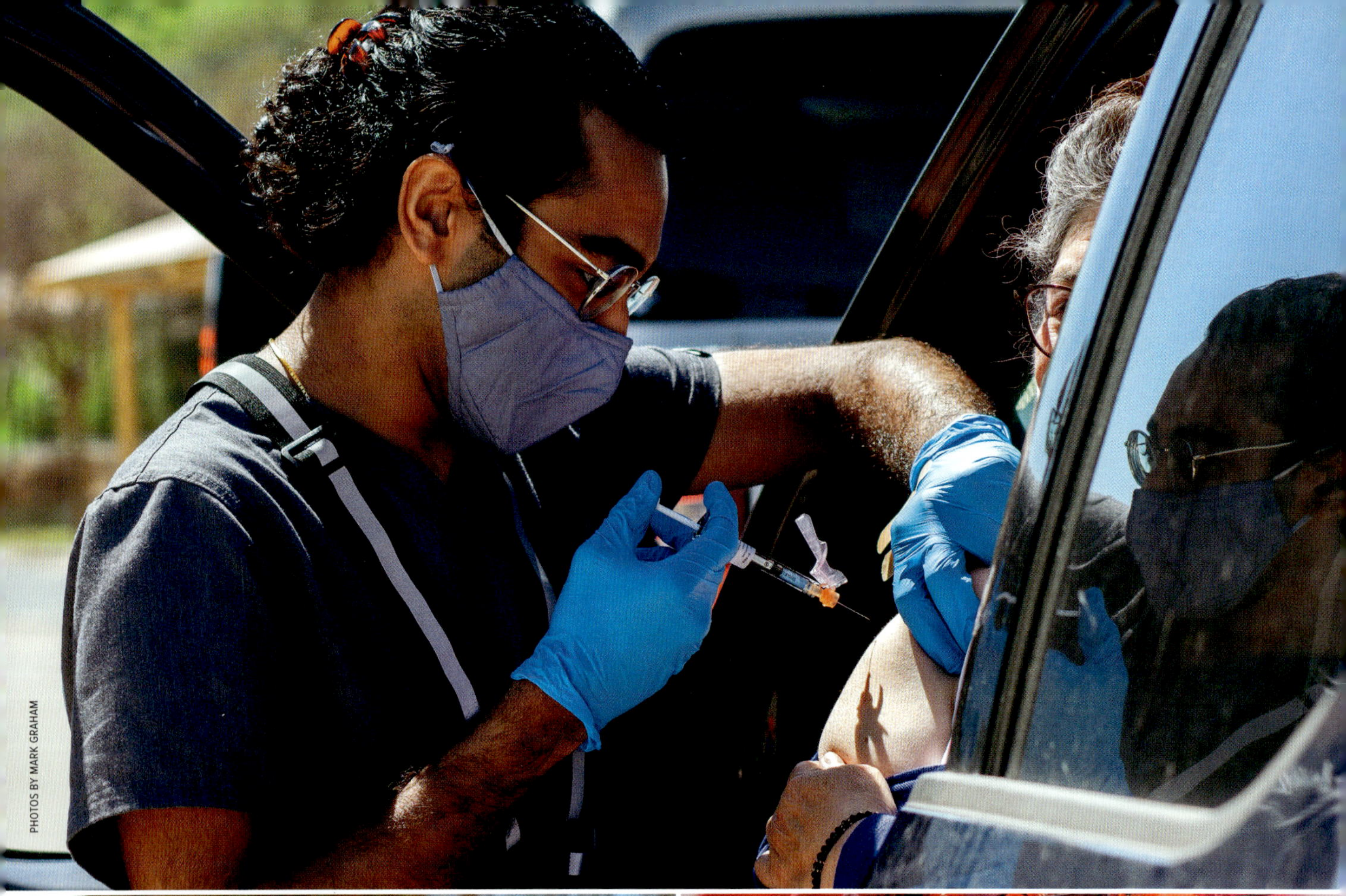

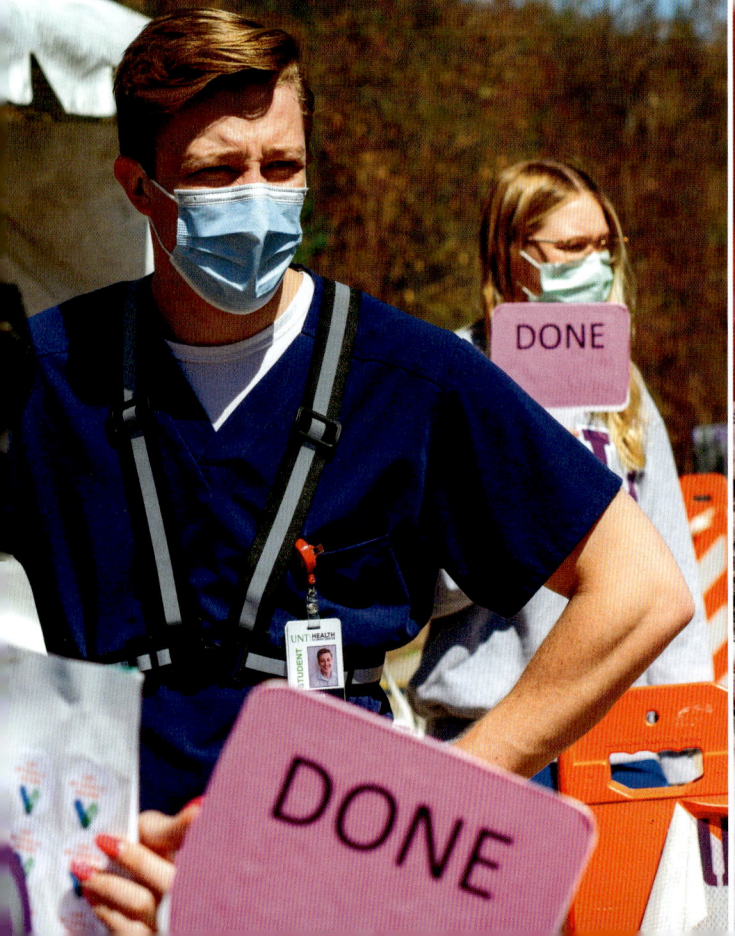

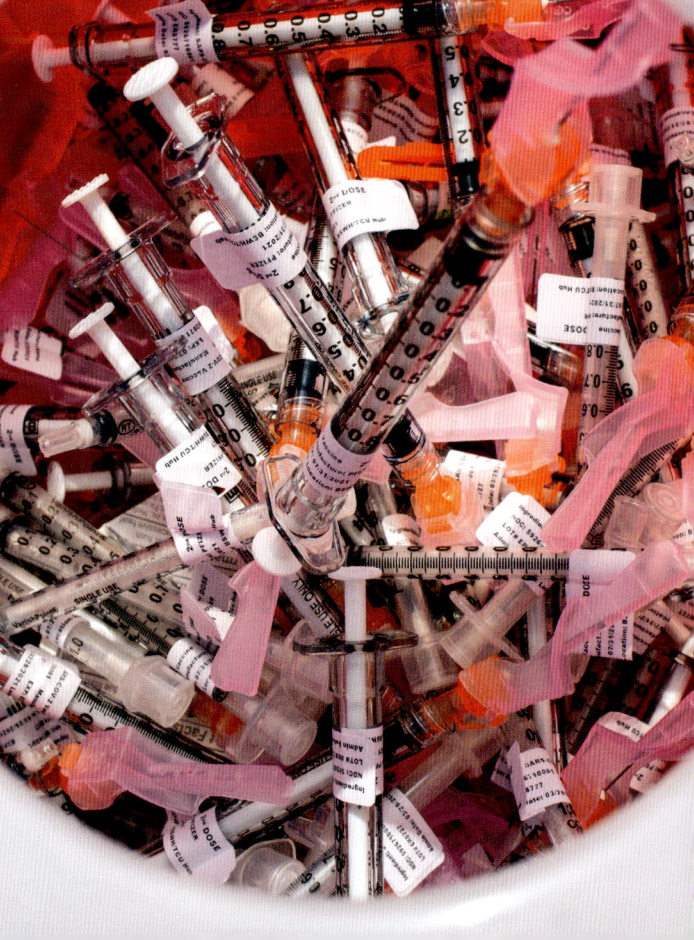

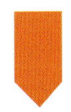

"Everyone in my class volunteered because it's such a unique opportunity at a really unique period of time."

Edmundo Esparza

worried about misinformation," said Shah, who during the winter grieved the loss of a close family friend to Covid-19.

He and his peers gave up parts of several weekends to vaccinate members of the community at a Fort Worth hospital and at TCU's Amon G. Carter Stadium.

"Part of the mission of this school is to play a positive role in community health," Losefsky said. "Administering the shot was one way we could all do that. People really seemed to appreciate what we were doing for them."

One Saturday in February 2021, Esparza spent the morning in Fort Worth's Northside and Diamond Hill neighborhoods registering residents of the largely Hispanic communities for the Covid shot. He then did a five-hour shift on the Baylor Scott & White All Saints campus, vaccinating people in cars as they wended their way through the parking lot.

"Everyone in my class volunteered because it's such a unique opportunity at a really unique period of time," said Esparza, who estimated he administered 80-100 vaccines in one afternoon. Improving the quality of life in Fort Worth had become a passion for the affable El Pasoan. He'd spearheaded a back-to-school drive six months earlier, collecting supplies for children living in the Como and Stop Six neighborhoods, in addition to Northside and Diamond Hill. Kruse helped him deliver boxes of crayons, paper and glue.

"To get all of these donations during the

pandemic was incredible," Esparza said. "It's also one of the great things about this school, that they let you run with an idea."

In their respective roles as vice president and president of the Latino Medical Student Association, he and Avila worked with fellow Hispanic students to create a class in medical Spanish.

"It was like a garage band going pro," Avila said. "We were really excited when the school agreed to our proposal to make the class an elective for next year."

Kinard co-chaired the regional conference of the Minority Association of Pre-Medical Students, an organization that supports members of underrepresented minority communities in their pursuit of a medical school education. She also mentored undergraduate members of TCU's association chapter.

Leadership and service positions beefed up the students' résumés, something particularly important for anyone intent on pursuing competitive specialties such as dermatology or neurosurgery.

Losefsky served as the medical student community administrator for the American College of Surgeons. While holed up at home as a massive winter storm dumped ice and snow on North Texas in February 2021, she created *Jeopardy*-style questions for the group's springtime conference, virtual that year.

For nearly her entire time in medical school, she helped recruit area physicians to speak at class functions. These kinds of interactions with physicians

Clockwise from top: Shah administered a Covid-19 vaccine at a drive-thru clinic; Student volunteers gave hundreds of shots at clinics around Fort Worth; Kruse waited for another driver to pull up to be immunized against the severe effects of Covid-19.

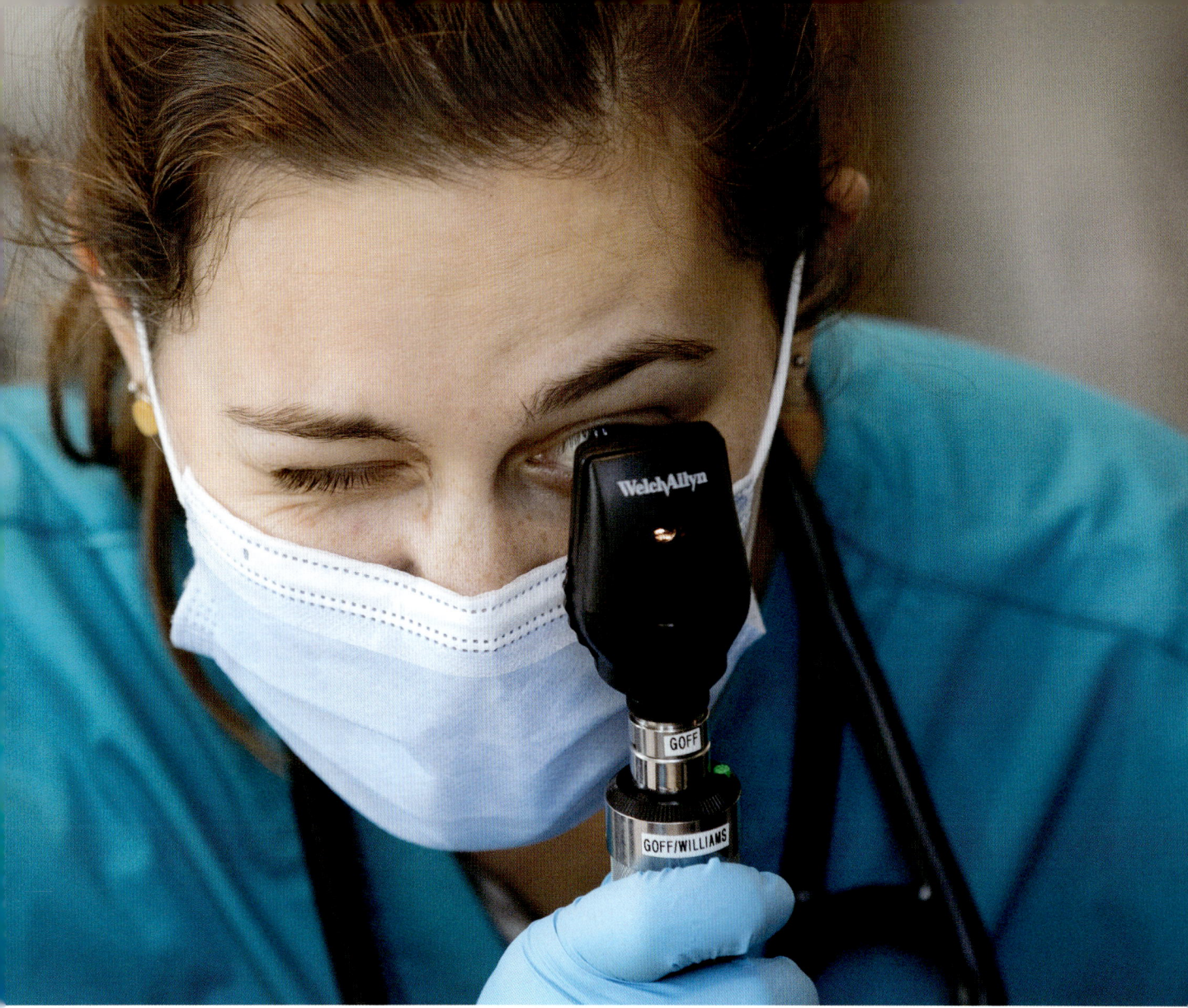

Losefsky practiced pediatrics exams in a classroom not long after the medical students returned to in-person instruction in September 2020.

who may provide networking, coaching and research opportunities can prove critical to a student's future.

"So much of medicine you can't learn from a book," said Losefsky, who also organized the school's surgery interest group. "Medicine is all about mentorship, especially once you transition to becoming a clinical med student."

* * *

Like most of her classmates, Losefsky felt the toll of long days and fast weeks, going from January to June 2021 without a break. She regularly sought out extra surgical shifts, meaning she might work at a hospital for 11 days in a row.

In the role of first assist, Losefsky spent hours with surgeons in the operating room, handing off surgical instruments during procedures large and small. She became adept at closing — sewing up incisions with tiny and precise stitches, the type of which varied depending on their location and use.

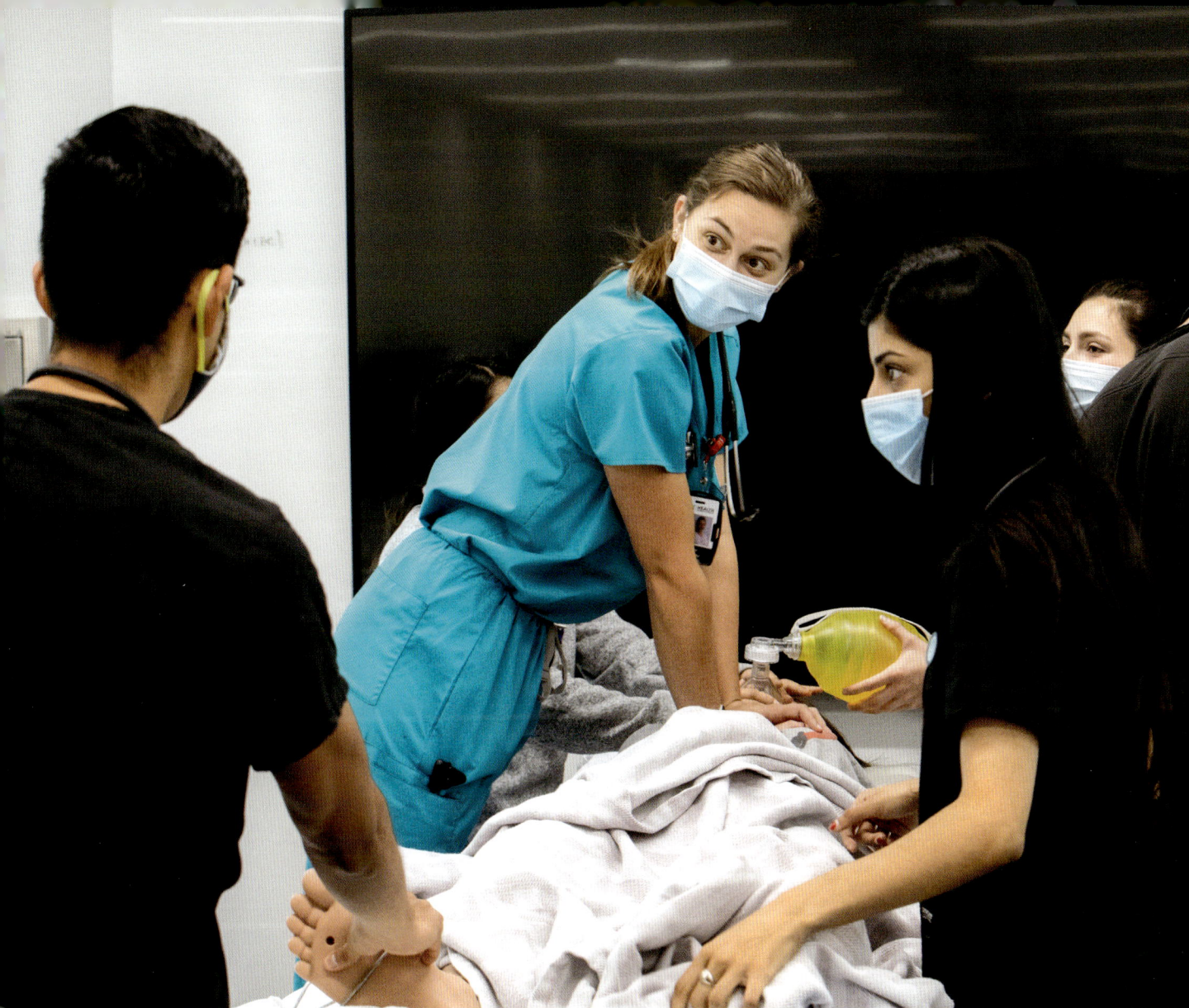

Losefsky ran a simulation of a coding patient alongside classmates including Sarah Cheema and Helena Kons.

Afterward she and the surgeon rounded on patients, hospital-speak for checking on them. While walking the hallways, faculty doctors quizzed her and her fellow students on how they might approach a particular case. They'd ask about anything from anatomy to what medications to prescribe to what steps to take in case of infection.

Physicians such as Rohan Jeyarajah emphasized the importance of broad learning that extended outside the students' intended areas of specialty.

Medical school is the only time doctors in the U.S. work in a range of disciplines.

Though Losefsky knew obstetrics wasn't her calling, she did fulfill her dream of catching a baby early in her second year. Before working nights at Baylor Scott & White All Saints Medical Center in October 2020, she bought a pair of black rain boots — the footwear of choice for most professionals in labor and delivery.

Midway into Losefsky's first week, she delivered a

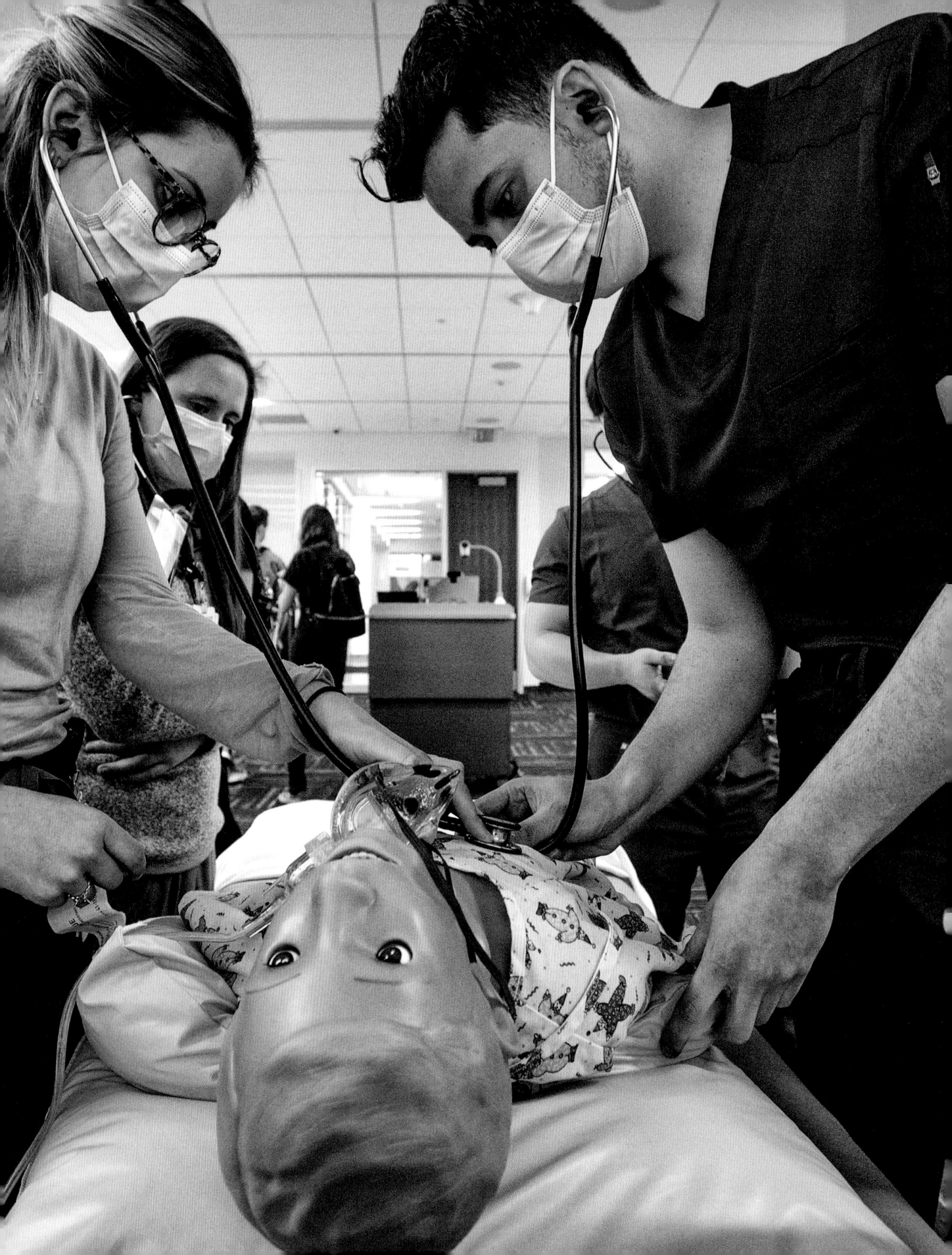

boy in the company of an attending physician and nurses. "I actually got a little teary," she said. "I was the first thing the baby saw."

Jeyarajah encouraged the students to embrace these varied experiences, some of which they might unexpectedly revisit in their careers. "I tell my students that whatever field they go into they'll end up seeing surgical patients," said the chair of the medical school's surgery department. "If you're a psychiatrist working in the psych ward, one of your patients will have appendicitis at some point."

Medical school becomes more demanding across the board in the second year, he said, something the students noticed as well.

If Losefsky planned to scrub in on surgeries, she typically devoted the evening beforehand to reviewing gross anatomy, studying the charts of upcoming cases and even sketching out procedures on paper to help her prepare.

In the absence of an impending surgery, she'd study for upcoming exams, often with online flashcards. "As a second-year, there is this press of time that I definitely didn't feel last year," she said. "I am always busy and always feeling like I could and should be doing more."

* * *

The competitive nature of residency placement added another layer of pressure to the students' experience as undergraduates in medical school.

"Residency is something you're always thinking about," Kruse said. "It's the big unknown."

Some feared missing out on certain residency programs because they hadn't yet picked a lane during the first half of medical school. The dean offered reassurance, saying that even third-year students had time to decide on specialties. "This is where their coaches and career advising can come in," Flynn said.

Residency programs look at applicants' scientific research, something each student must do as part of TCU's Scholarly Pursuit and Thesis project. Students choose areas of interest and begin working with mentors, typically in the first

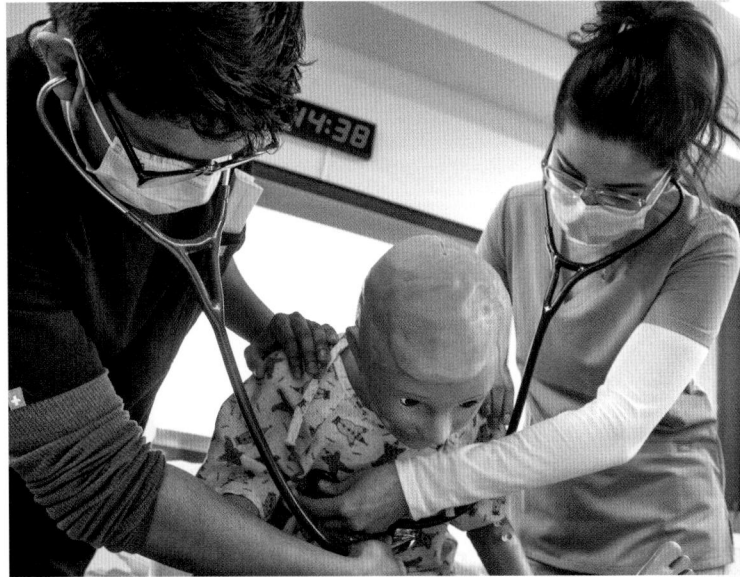

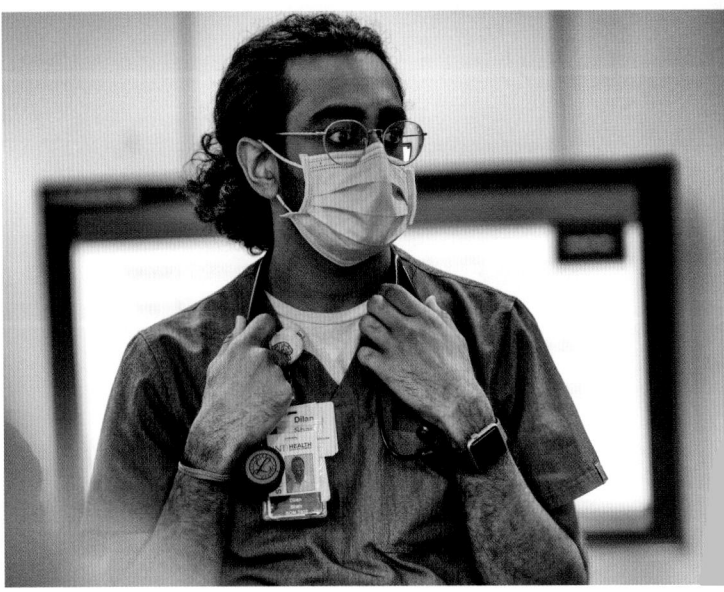

Left: From left, McKenna Chalman and Grace Newell, both of whom attended TCU as undergraduates, worked alongside Esparza to study lung and heart diseases with the help of a manikin.

Above: The Burnett School of Medicine emphasizes hands-on learning over traditional lectures. Avila, top, with Arman Fijany, and Shah, below, learned and practiced their skills under the watchful eyes of some 400 area physicians. By 2024, the faculty had grown to more than 1,400.

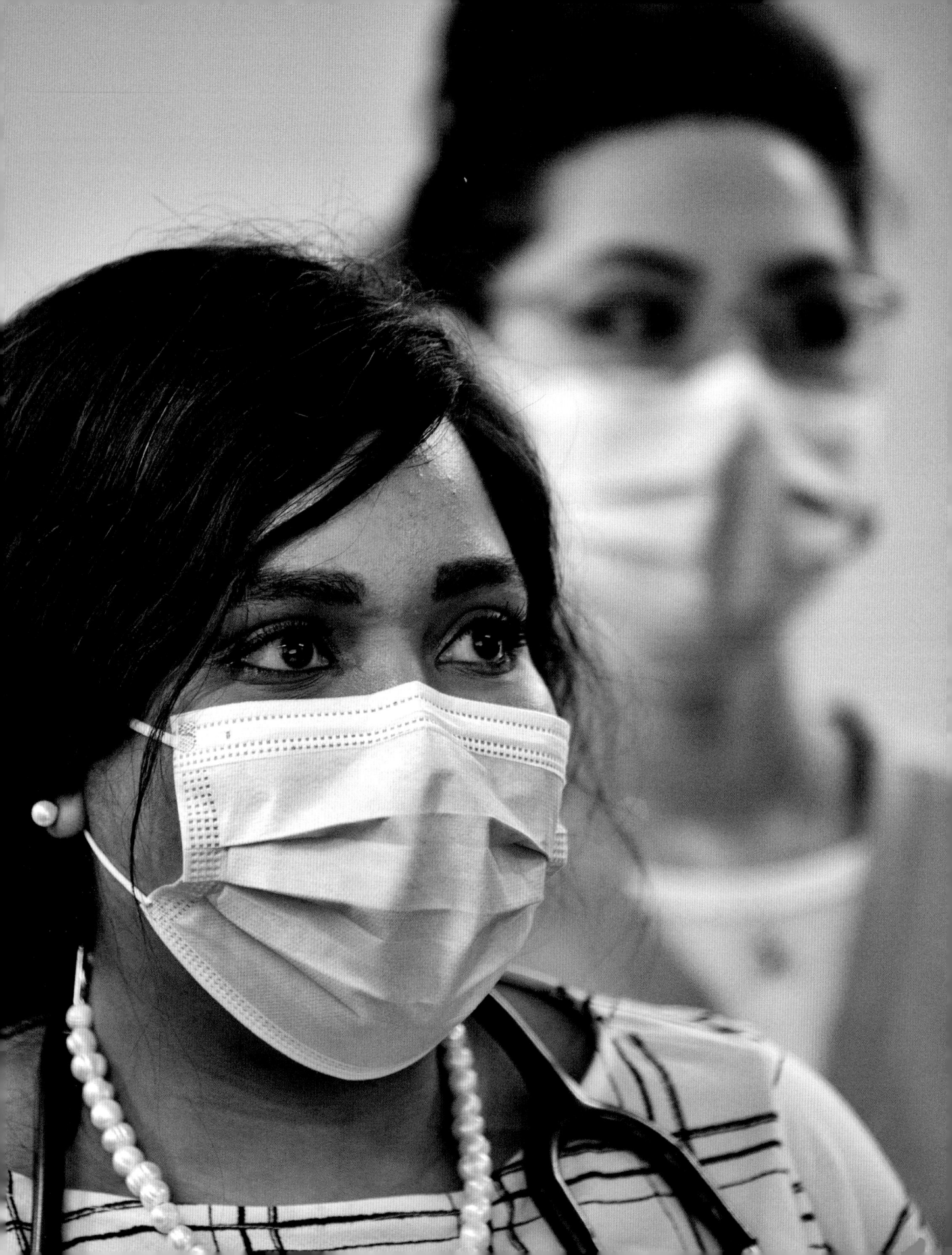

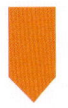

Kinard, Avila and their 56 classmates in Year 2 balanced research, real patient care and traditional medical academics while also learning empathy and communication skills at the Burnett School of Medicine.

year of school. Beyond the capstone project, graduation requirements include a presentation at a research symposium.

That was how a windowless lab on the first floor of Sid Richardson Physical Sciences Building on the east side of the TCU campus became Kinard's second home. There she performed experiments with graphene quantum dots, a nanomaterial that delivers chemotherapy drugs directly to cells.

"The more effective the delivery system, the smaller the amount of drugs that can be used," Kinard said.

During her time at the Burnett School of Medicine, Kinard was the only medical student on a team led by Anton Naumov, an assistant professor of physics whom she described as a powerhouse in the field.

"The goal is that they will have publishable research by the end of medical school, but the Scholarly Pursuit and Thesis project helps with other skills, like time management," said Michael Bernas, director of the program. "Just like when they are professionals, they have to find ways to do their research outside of official clinical duties."

* * *

Many of the students encountered something akin to the sophomore slump. The relentless pace of school during the second year, coupled with gloomy bouts of weather, seemed to affect the collective mood of the class in the winter and spring. The Covid crisis didn't help.

Nor did ongoing worries about money. Many took out $80,000 in loans for Year 2. Tuition for the 2020-21 academic year totaled $60,318, though a grant from the school along with a scholarship from a donor trimmed some of that cost.

"A lot of us have fallen into a pit of despair because of how hard this has been," said Shah, who did feel reinvigorated that April after a Zoom meeting with some Harvard medical students. The Burnett School of Medicine organized the session so the upperclassmen could give encouragement to the TCU students. That mentorship continued with another panel session in June.

Shah and his peers mentored the school's 60 first-year medical students. The Class of 2024 started all-online in July 2020 and remained mostly virtual the entire year, with minimal coursework and few exams in person.

Upon hearing that many of the second-year students felt fatigued, Flynn expressed little surprise.

"Covid sapped a lot of energy, though I don't want to use that as a scapegoat," he said. "Clerkship is the toughest year for medical students because of the pressure. You have to be evaluated, and you want to excel."

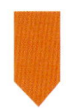

> **"There's a gravity and weight because I'm not just learning something that's rhetorical or theoretical anymore. This is someone's life, and that settles on your soul."**
>
> Quinn Losefsky

* * *

Esparza weighed his options about specialties during his second year while rebounding from an emotionally draining spring. Frequent workouts at the TCU gym helped, as did focusing on how far he'd come in his medical education.

"I don't ever worry about going into a patient room now and talking to someone," he said. "I know I know how to communicate with empathy and compassion."

Esparza also believed the staff in hospitals and clinics treated them more like fourth-year medical students, another confidence booster.

Losefsky entered medical school already knowing a number of local physicians from her three years working as a scribe while an undergraduate at TCU. Starting in 2017, she'd documented information and conversations in the emergency room at Texas Health Harris Methodist Hospital Fort Worth.

As a medical student, she learned that "the more time you spend in the OR with a doctor, the more you can anticipate their needs." Losefsky also spent hours practicing the use of both hands during surgery. She mastered tying knots while wearing two layers of gloves covered in blood.

"I'm at a point now where I can grab instruments for the surgeons before they ask," she said. "I always want to make myself as useful to them as I can."

Over the course of the year, physicians directed the students to take on more responsibilities, such as interviewing patients, writing up chart notes and doing supervised procedures.

"This is the hardest I've ever worked," Kruse said, "but working with patients is definitely better than sitting in a lecture hall."

Dealing with patients could present its own set of challenges, as Avila discovered.

"I've experienced more full-on direct racism in the past two years than I have in my entire life," she said.

As the country turned its attention to the crisis at the border with Mexico, a patient locked eyes with her and said, "I know you people need somewhere to go" before unleashing a rant about migrants. "It baffles me that there are people who truly think it's OK to verbalize these things to someone's face and be that offensive," Avila said.

Kinard once feared she might be subjected to overt racism in Texas. While that hadn't transpired by the end of her second year, she had encountered subtle actions or comments directed at people of color. "Sometimes I'm assumed to be other races because I look ambiguous," Kinard said, noting she'd been repeatedly asked "What are you?" or "Where are you really from?"

She learned to look beyond such behavior. "Sometimes it feels like death by a thousand paper

Burnett School of Medicine students train for a range of emergency situations.

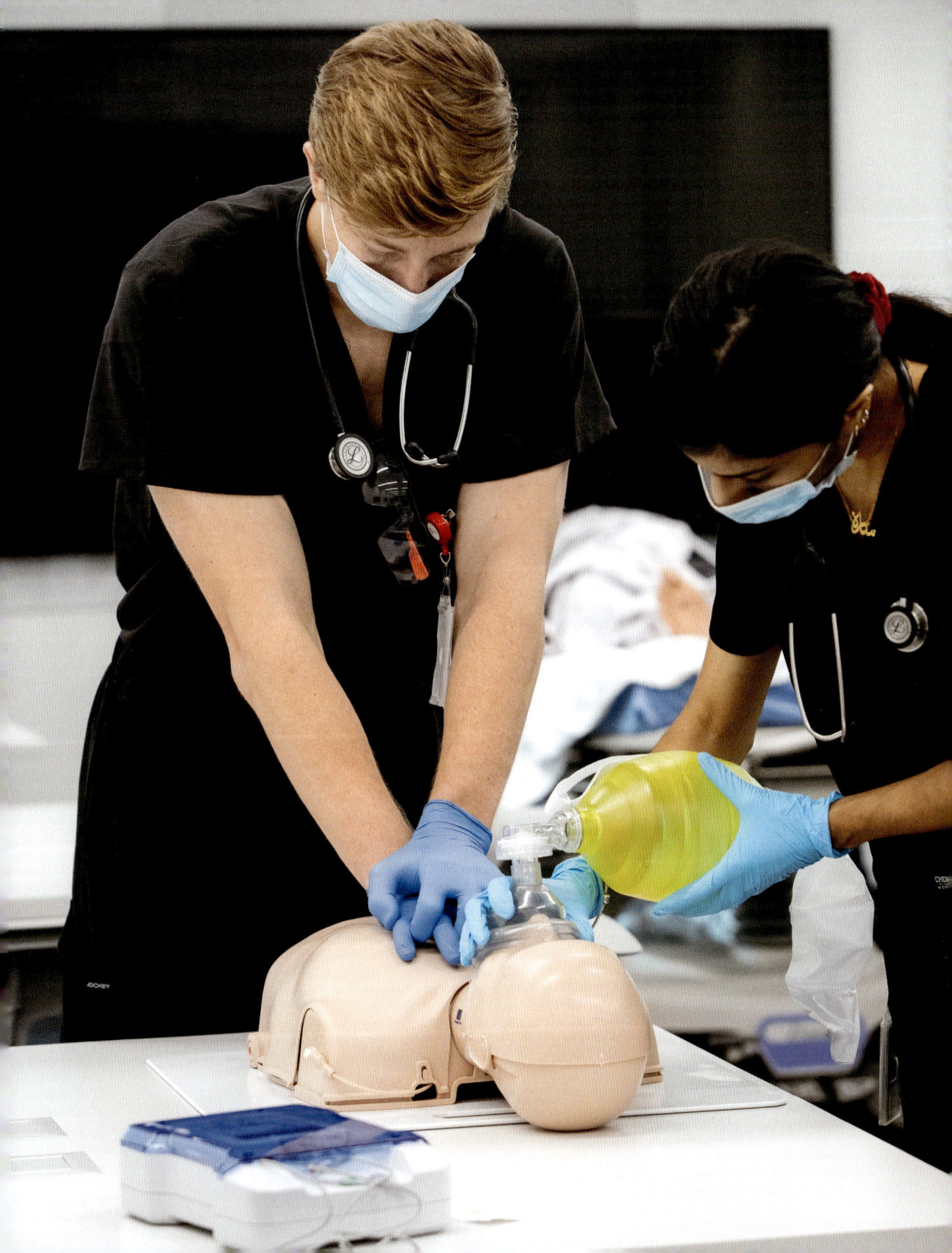

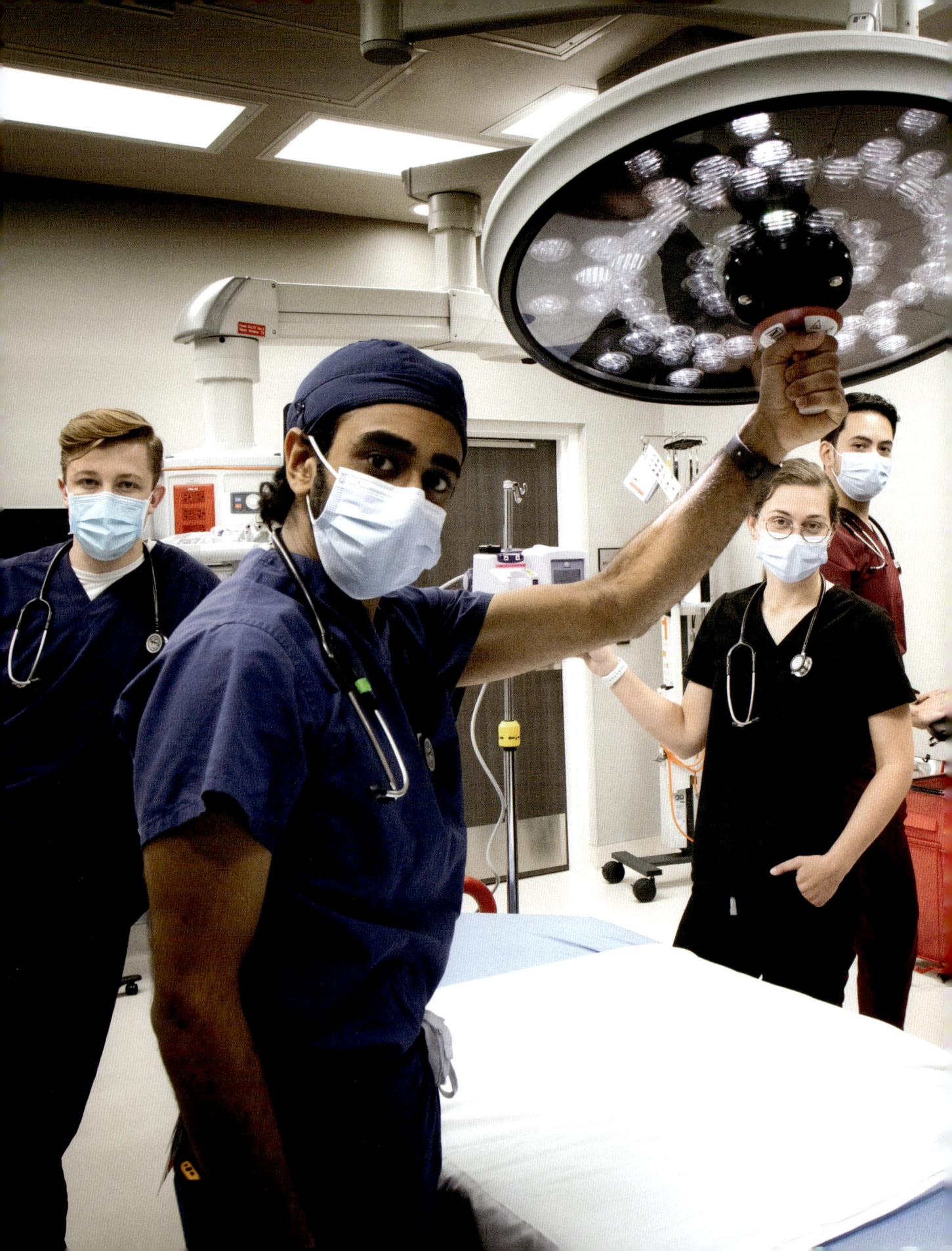

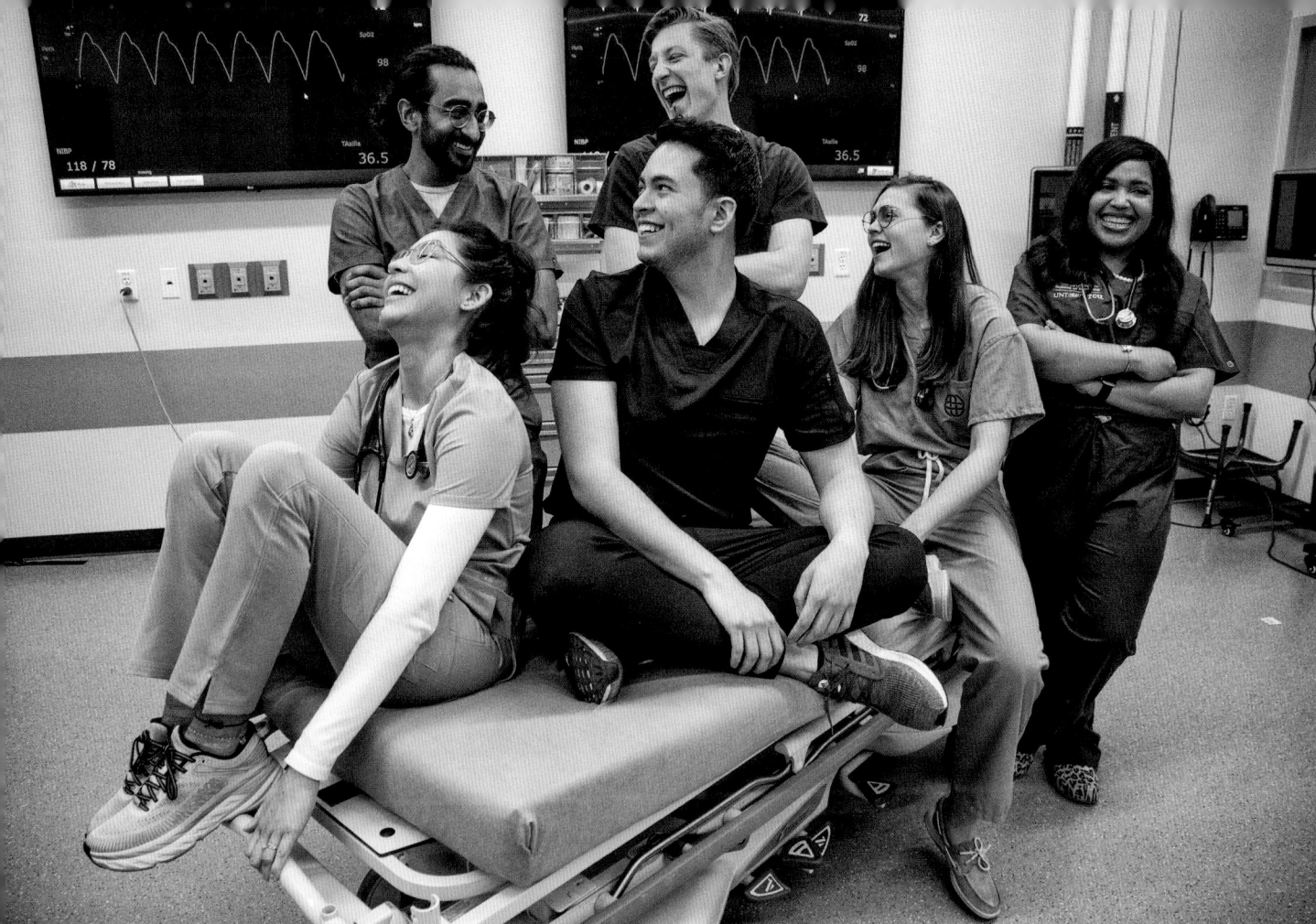

Above: The *TCU Magazine* six shared a laugh toward the end of the high-stakes second year of medical school. Left: Kruse, Shah, Losefsky and Esparza took precautions from Covid while diving back into work at area hospitals and continuing their medical education.

cuts, but I work hard to put it out of my mind," she said. "If I am upset, then I can't study for the rest of the night."

One of Avila's mentors counseled her that she always has the right to walk away. "That was very empowering, the idea I could find someone else to treat the patient," Avila said. "They can choose to be nasty, and I can choose not to take it."

Losefsky, meanwhile, gained new appreciation for patients who trust their surgeons to inflict harm on their bodies in the service of healing them. "I'm literally manipulating their unconscious body, something that's so personal and so intimate," she said. "I always feel like I need to work to earn that."

She'd suctioned clots off brains and kept a

liter of blood from blocking a surgeon's view of the spine for 6½ hours. That second year, she saw more hernias and infected gallbladders than she could count. She also watched patients die.

"There's a gravity and weight because I'm not just learning something that's rhetorical or theoretical anymore," she said. "This is someone's life, and that settles on your soul."

Some of the patients and procedures kept her up at night, but an abiding passion for the work — plus the promise of Starbucks — made her bound out of bed before dawn, ready for whatever the day held.

"It can be exhausting," she said, "but I truly feel like this is what I was born to do." 🍃

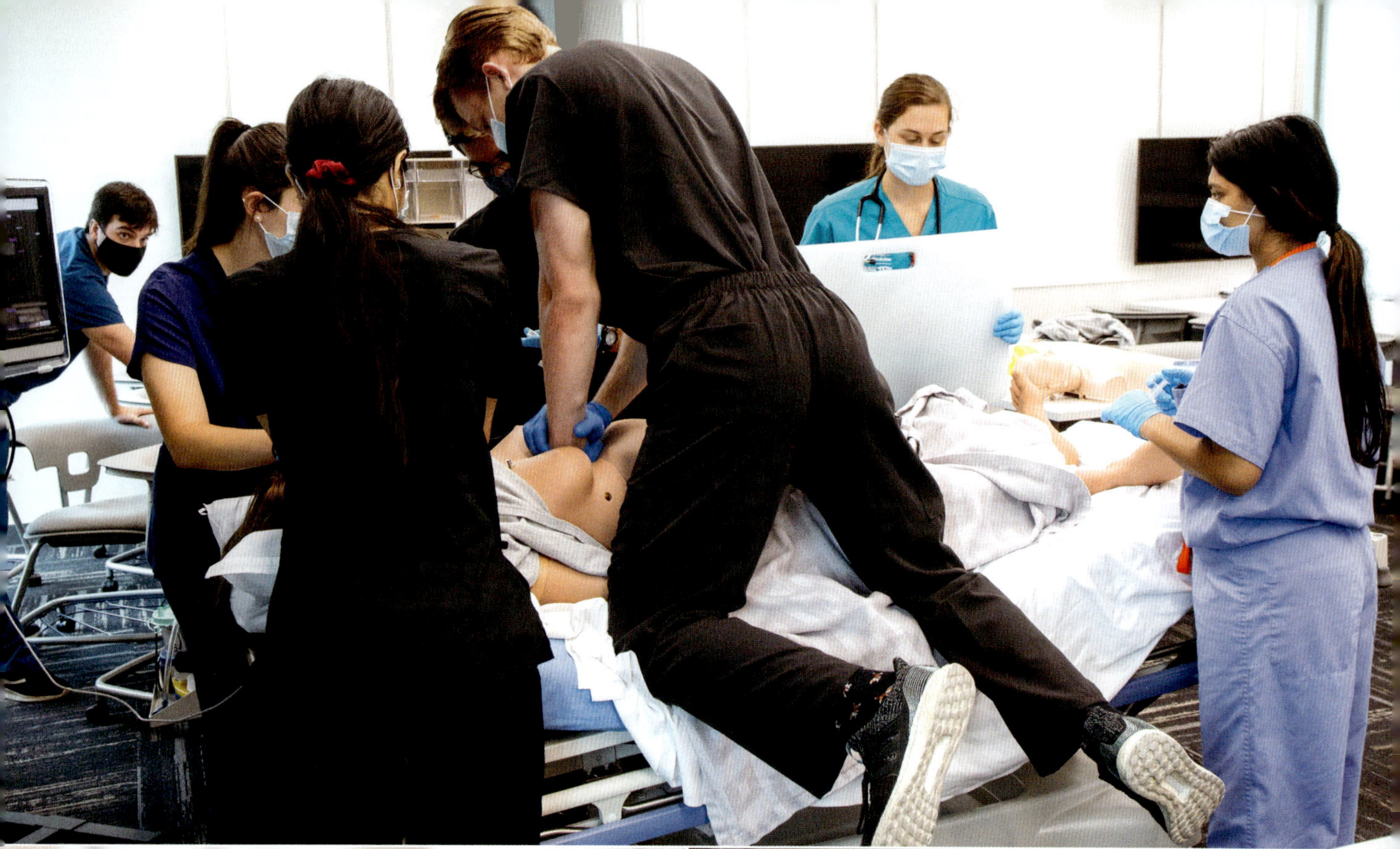

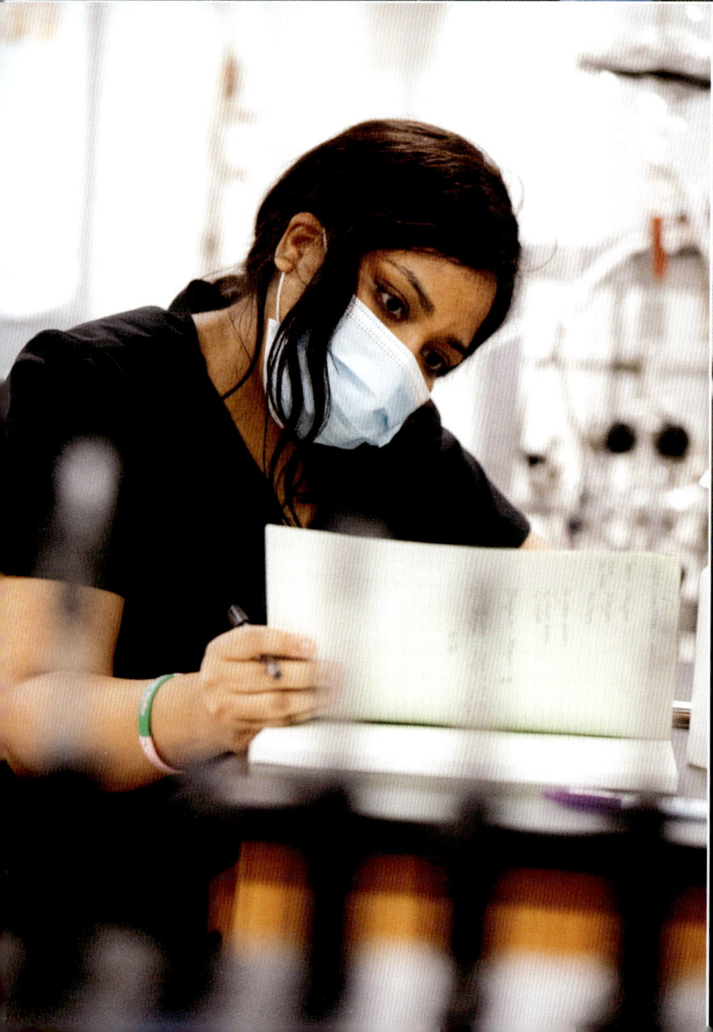

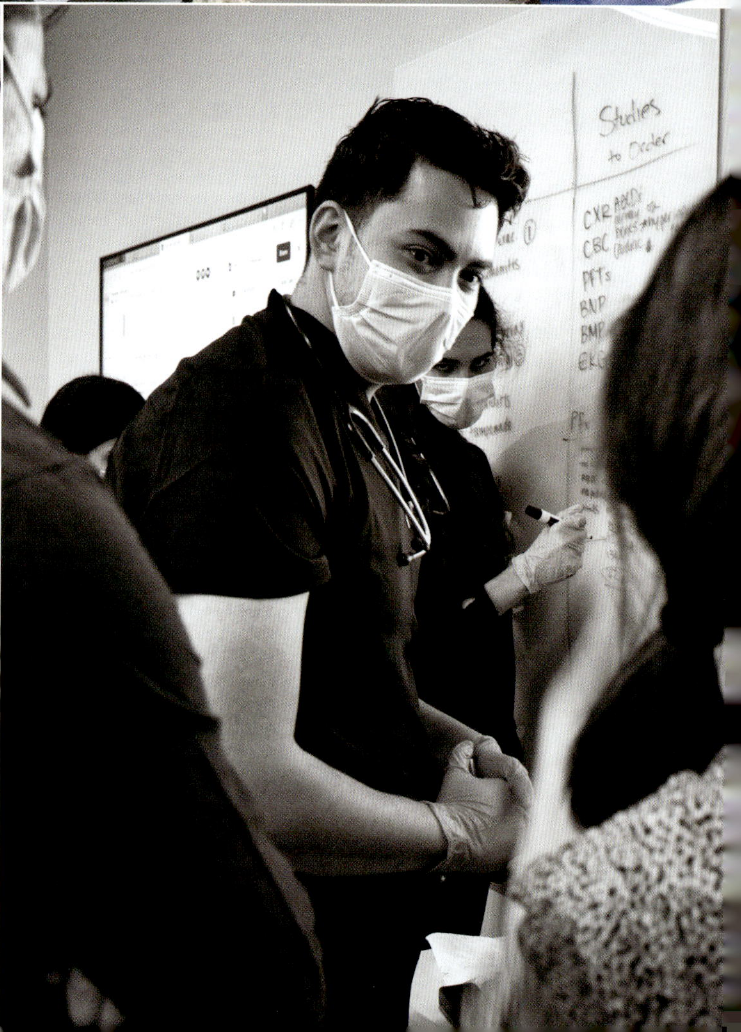
Studies
to Order
CXR
CBC
PFTs
BNP
BMP

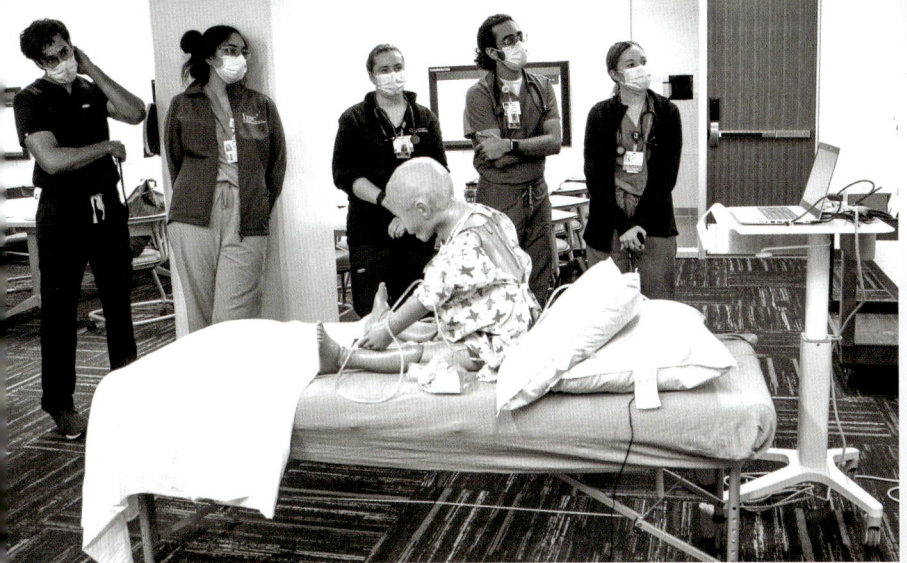

Opposite page, clockwise from top:

Kruse coordinated the response of his team, which included Losefsky, during a simulated crisis.

Esparza worked on clinical and communication skills simultaneously.

Kinard was the only medical student on the team studying nanotechnology in Anton Naumov's physics lab.

This page, from top:

Students from left, Ruthvik Allala, Kavneet Kaur, Sam Evans, Shah and Rachel Rice listened to instructions during a clinical skills class.

Shah attended a Zoom class to learn about admitting patients to the hospital.

Kruse studied a holographic anatomical model using a HoloLens 2 headset.

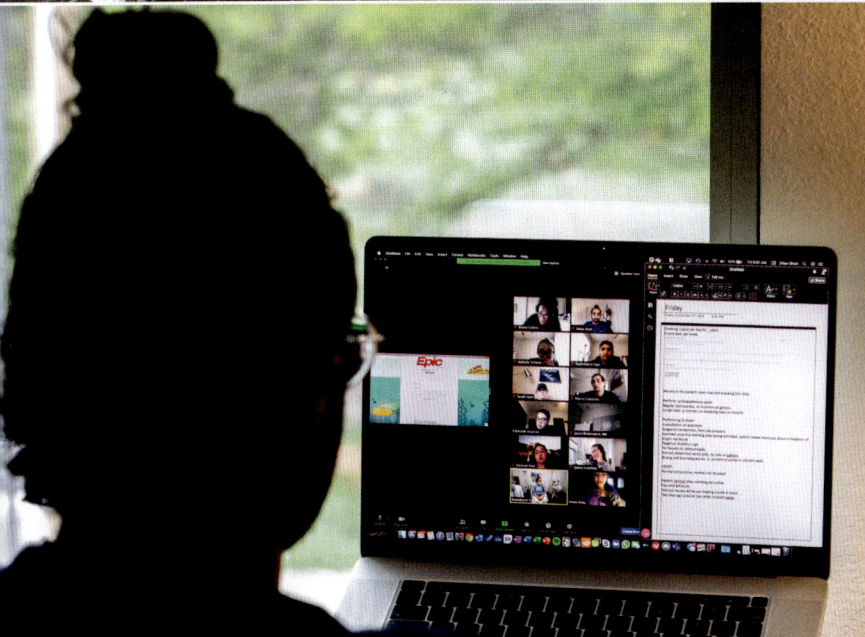

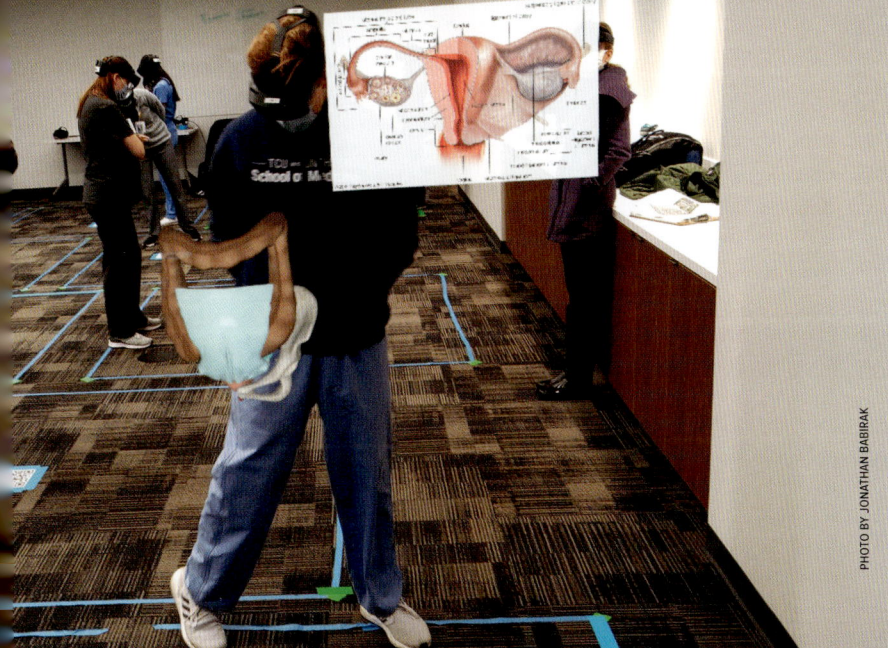

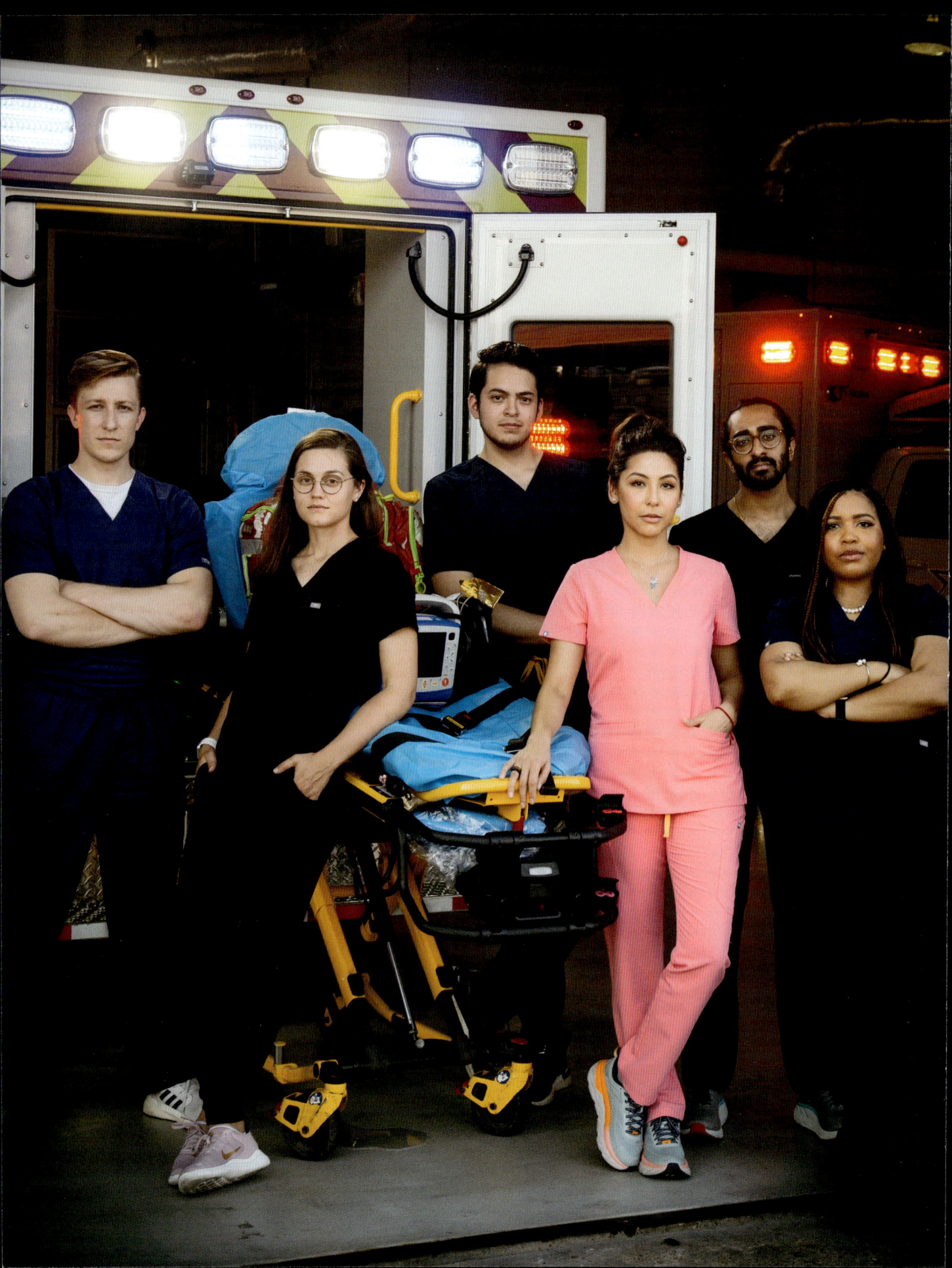

YEAR THREE

2021-22

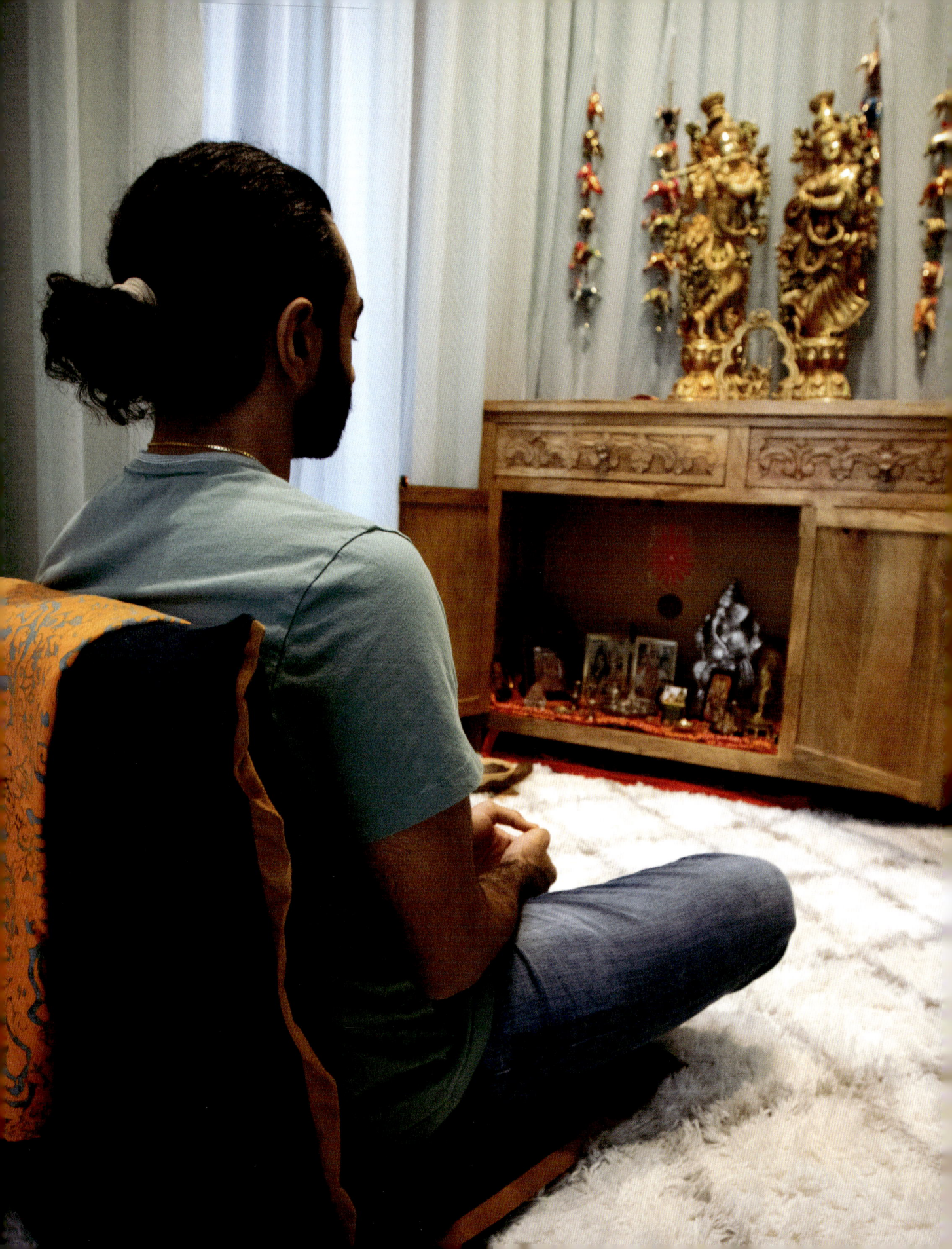

High Hopes

Turmoil in the U.S. and abroad became an unrelenting backdrop to the third year of medical school for the Class of 2023. Russia invaded Ukraine, its democratic neighbor to the west, in February 2022. Extreme heat, wildfires and drought roiled much of the U.S. as undocumented migrant crossings at the southern border topped a record 2.76 million for the fiscal year.

In May 2022, the U.S. surpassed 1 million deaths attributed to Covid-19.

That month, the Texas Department of State Health Services warned that every primary care specialty would see shortages within a decade, particularly the areas of psychiatry, pediatrics, family medicine, OB-GYN and internal medicine. At the same time, medical school applications across the country hit new highs. The Association of American Medical Colleges reported that applications soared by 17.8 percent for the 2021-22 school year, with underrepresented groups leading the surge.

More than 22,000 students in the U.S. began medical school in the fall semester of 2021, including the addition of 60 more to the Anne Burnett Marion School of Medicine. Thirty-five percent of the Class of 2025 came from Texas. The average age of the incoming students — 13 TCU graduates included — was 24, with the class evenly split between men and women.

Twenty-five percent of the new students had already attained graduate degrees in areas ranging from nursing practice and biomedical science to physiology and accounting. A full 70 percent of the class identified with at least one of three school-defined diversity domains: race/ethnicity, LGBTQ and socioeconomic limitation.

* * *

Students in the Class of 2023 entered the third year of medical school with a singular goal: to achieve the highest possible score on the Step 1 and Step 2 tests. Like all would-be doctors, they had to pass three United States Medical Licensing Examinations. The first two, which they sat for during the third year of school, carried the added pressure of helping determine the course of postgraduate education.

In advance of the Step 1, Dilan Shah spent hours meditating in his childhood bedroom, working to tame anxiety related to the test, while his housemate Quinn Losefsky adhered to a rigorous study schedule she'd designed at the first of the year.

By the time he took the make-or-break test in mid-November 2021, Jonas Kruse had achieved a 650-day streak of quizzing himself with online flashcards. Studying with that level of intensity had become as much a part of his routine, his wife said, as brushing his teeth or walking their dogs.

Charna Kinard and Ive Avila sat for the exam a few weeks later, after two months of studying 14 hours a day.

While Edmundo Esparza was taking the Step 1 in November, his computer at his test site froze, disrupting his progress and leaving him rattled. He

Dilan Shah relied on his meditation practice to stay focused during preparation for the all-important Step 1 exam.

"This is the most important test of your career. How you score dictates everything from what type of residency program you can apply to, to what kind of hospital and city you'll end up in."

Edmundo Esparza

described the exam as pushing him to the edge of burnout. "This is the most important test of your career," he said. "How you score dictates everything from what type of residency program you can apply to, to what kind of hospital and city you'll end up in.

"It's that big of a deal."

* * *

The students faced a range of challenges in Year 3, some of which felt overwhelming at times.

Esparza had endured an unsettling start to his third year at TCU. During his MBA program at the University of Texas at El Paso, he'd gone to the emergency room with searing pain from kidney stones. He carried the debt from that hospital visit, plus two others he'd made while uninsured, into medical school.

Though the Burnett School of Medicine discourages students from holding jobs, Esparza drove on occasion for the ride-share services Uber or Lyft when money was tight. But he relied on loans to fund living expenses like rent and food in addition to the biggest expense: tuition.

Esparza had managed to pay off two outstanding medical debts when unbeknownst to him the remaining unpaid debt was sold to another collection

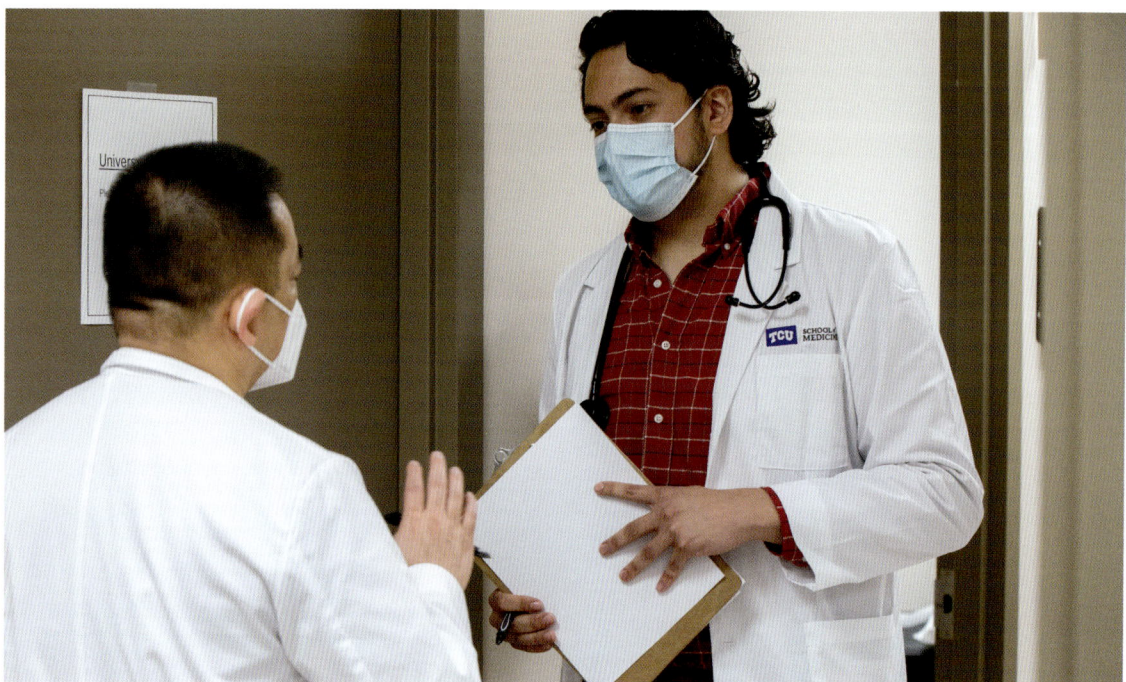

Above: Edmundo Esparza shadowed Dr. Khuong Phan at Mansfield Medical Associates. Right: Esparza conducted a patient interview and exam on Gisele Paviani.

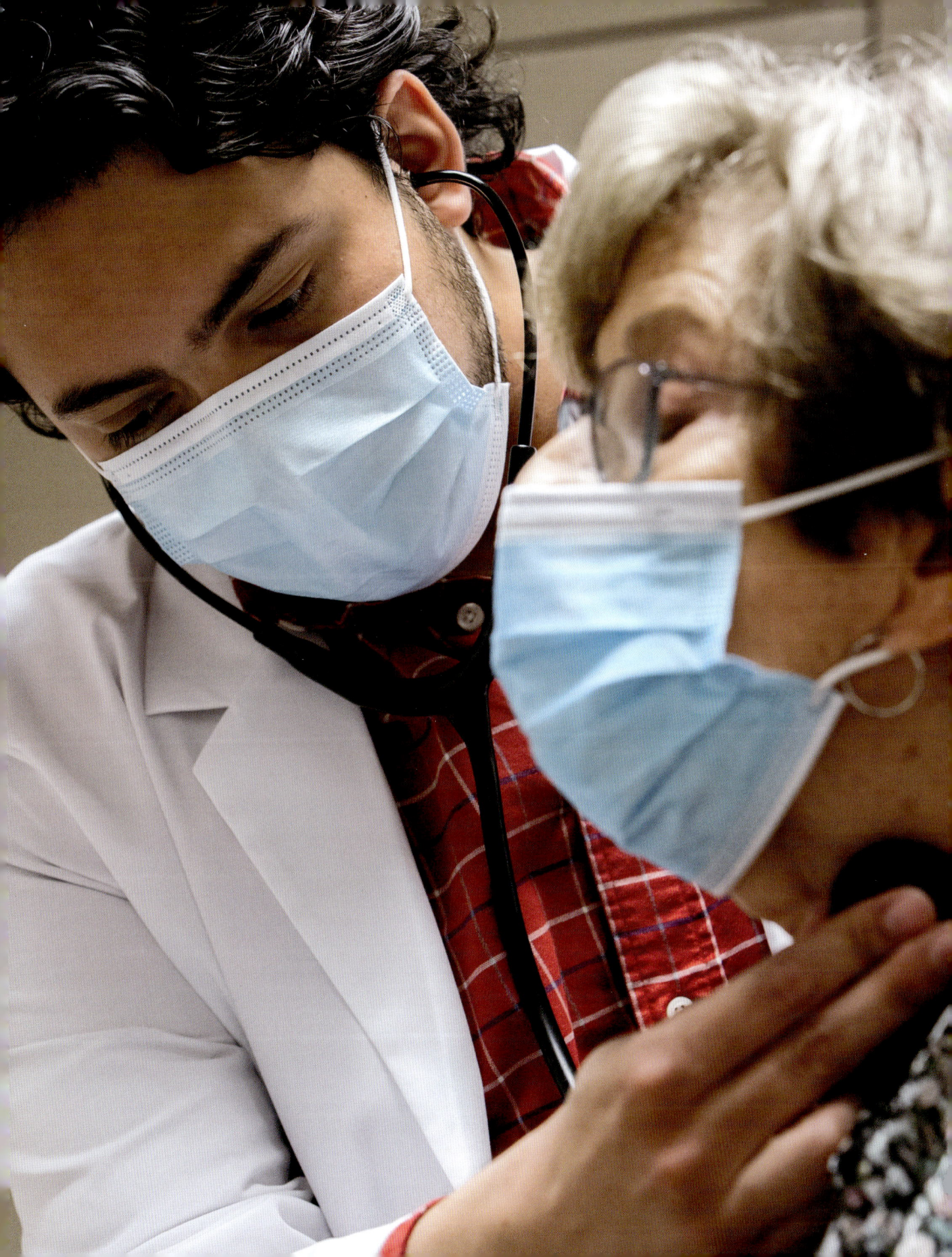

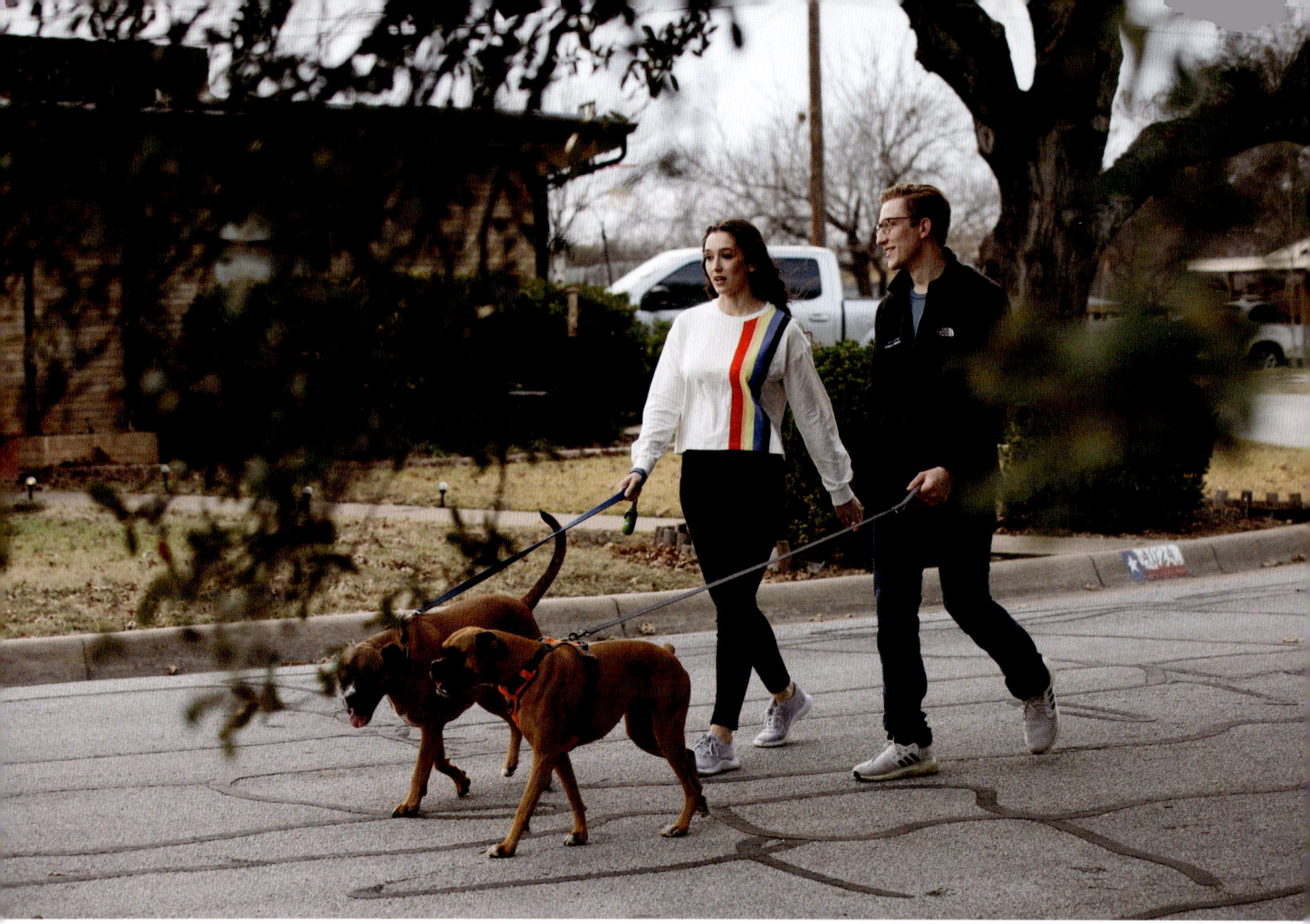

Jonas Kruse and his wife, Anabel, took their energetic rescue boxers, Harley and Hank, on frequent walks around their Fort Worth neighborhood.

agency. When the debt hit his credit report as a new loan, Esparza was automatically denied his $40,000 GradPlus Loan for the 2021-22 academic year.

"It's killing me," he said in the first few days of the third year of medical school, when his fate was up in the air. "There's a chance I might have to take a gap year now if it's not straightened out in time."

Despite several deans rallying to support him, Esparza's appeals were denied. In late July, one of his brothers stepped in to pay off the debt. The original total was $2,500, but the Esparzas settled it for $1,400.

Worries about money swirled in his mind throughout medical school. By the end of his third year, he had amassed $240,000 in student loans, a figure that topped $300,000 by graduation.

At the start of Kruse's second year of medical school, his maternal grandmother died in Orange County, California. Not long after taking the Step 1 exam in November 2021, he flew west for a week to help care for his widowed grandfather. He was part of the family's decision to move the 94-year-old into an assisted living facility in January 2022, where he continued to thrive more than two years later.

"He'll tell anyone who listens that his advice for a long life is ice cream, wine, Fig Newtons and a good marriage," Kruse said.

Losefsky signed up to take the Step 1 exam only to learn that her mother's prophylactic double mastectomy had been scheduled for that same early November day. Her mom carries the mutation in the

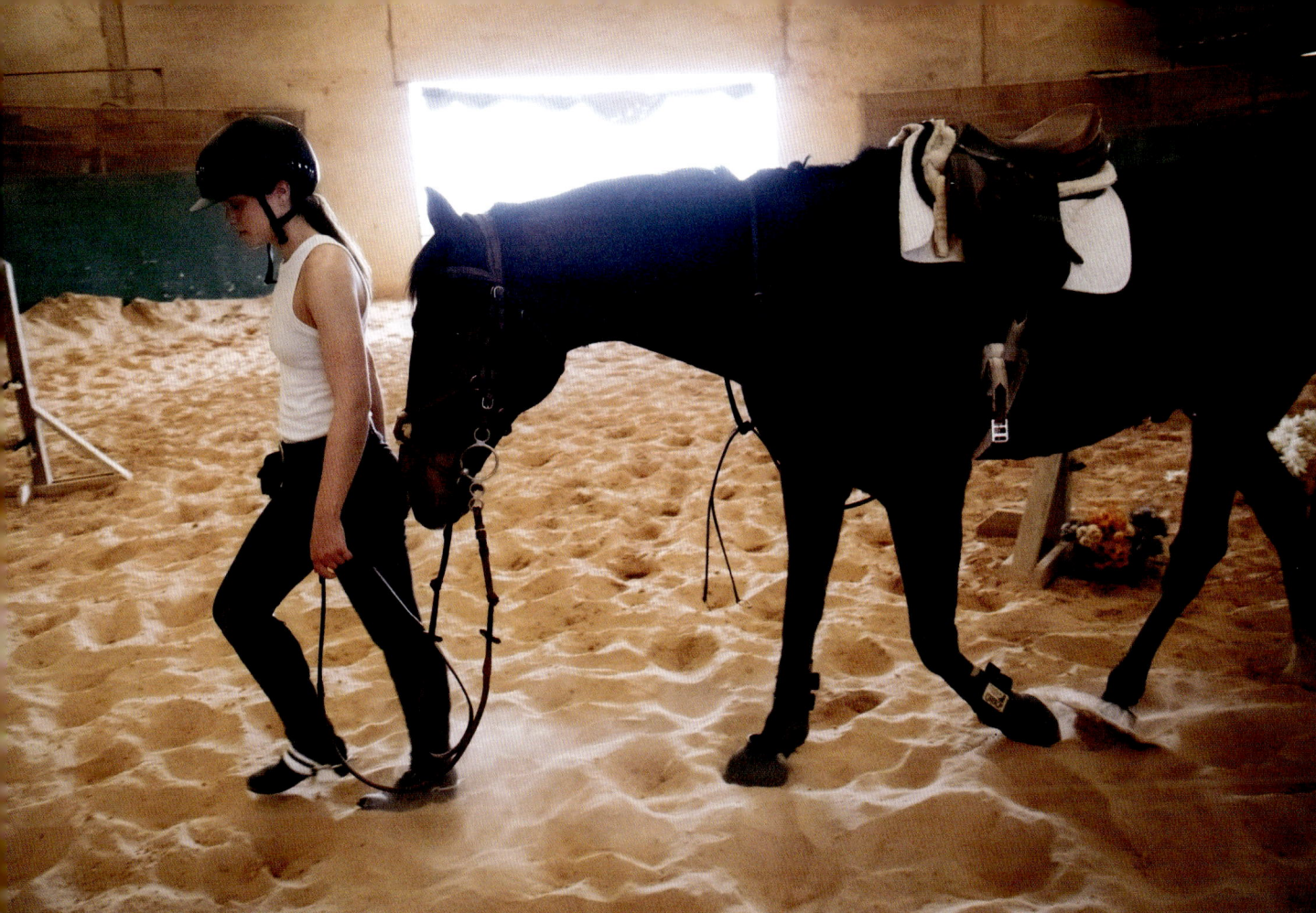

A lifelong horsewoman, Quinn Losefsky took riding lessons throughout medical school.

BRCA1 gene, giving her an 85 percent chance of getting breast cancer. While still in high school, Losefsky learned that she, too, had inherited the gene.

"My mom's surgery was something I didn't expect to worry about on the most impactful and stressful day of the year," she said. Since students could take the exam anywhere in the country, she chose to sit for the Step 1 in Austin. After finishing that afternoon, Losefsky drove straight to the hospital, where she learned that her mother's five-hour surgery, which included the meticulous removal of breast tissue as well as total reconstruction, had gone perfectly.

While most of her classmates were still studying for the critical test, Losefsky put her education to use, changing drains, managing her mom's pain while cooking nutritious meals. Any fears she had about the timing evaporated three weeks later when her test results arrived.

"The relief at doing well was overwhelming," Losefsky said.

Avila, who spent most of 2021 pregnant, dealt with the medical community in Austin in the summer of 2021, but with a far less positive outcome. Right as Avila was finishing her second year of medical school, her 80-year-old maternal grandmother called to say she couldn't feel her legs. Avila phoned an uncle to tell him to rush her grandmother to the emergency room.

Avila's grandmother had a blood clot. When surgery was scheduled for a week later, Avila, who was nearing the end of her first trimester at the time,

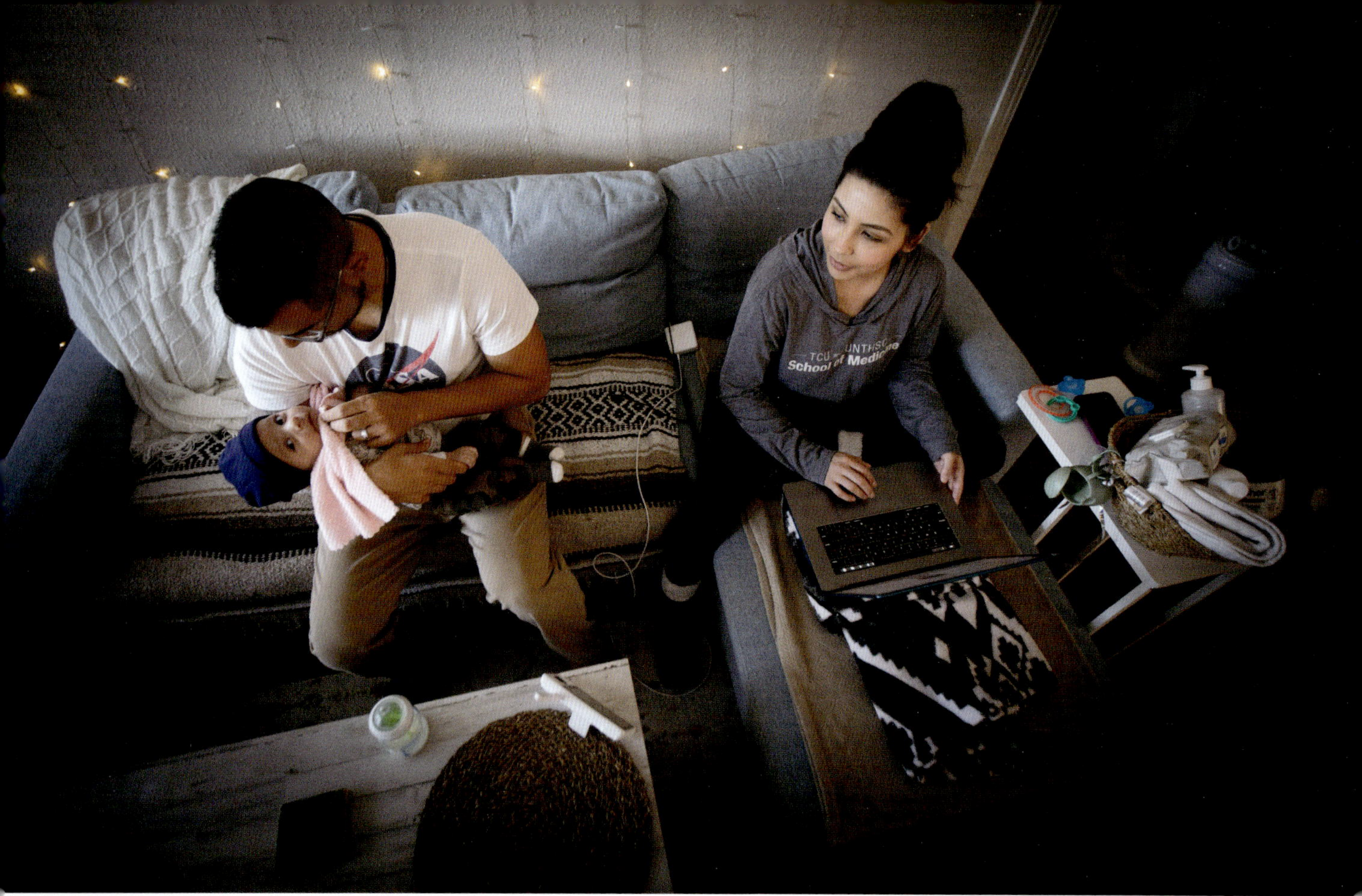

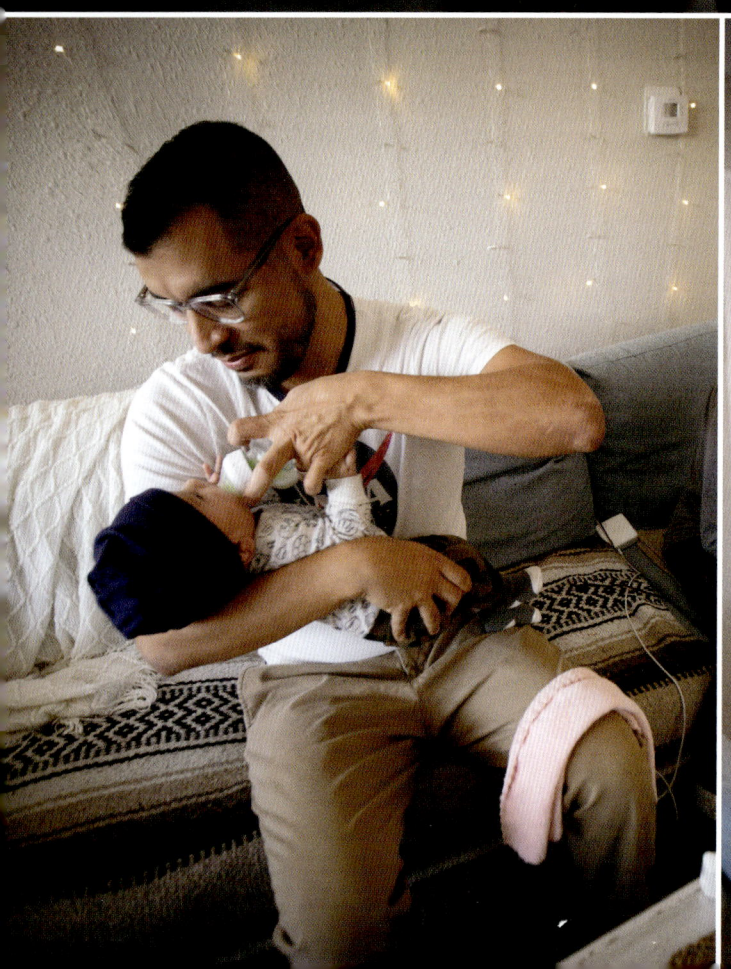
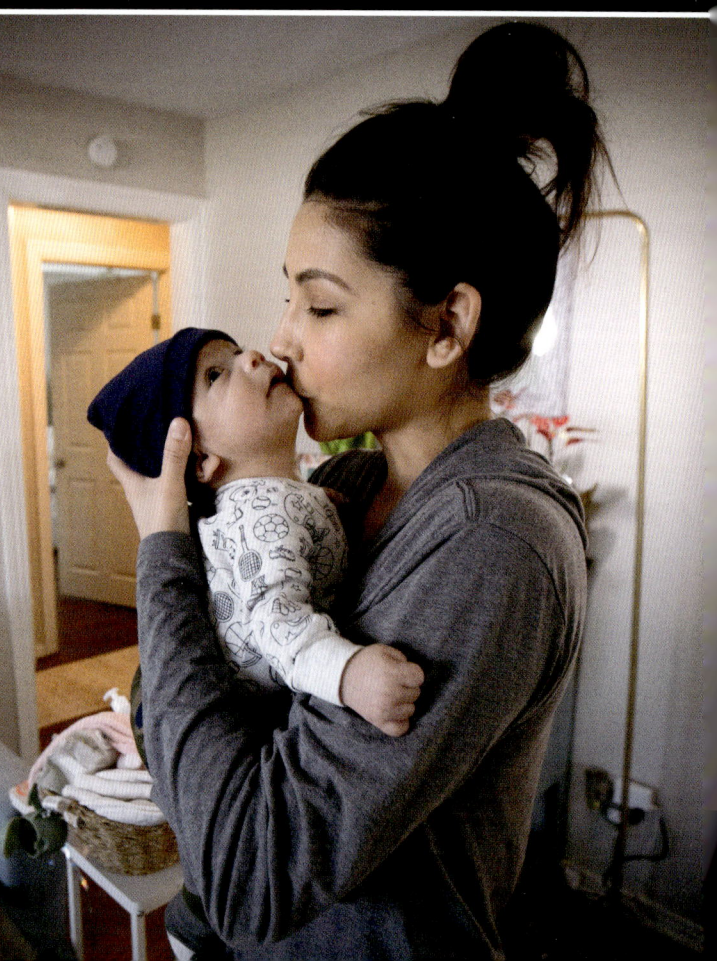

successfully lobbied her grandmother's primary care physician to move up the procedure.

Following surgery, her grandmother, who spoke only Spanish, complained of a terrible headache. The attending nurse treated her with Tylenol. The nurse called security on Avila's family as they begged her to help their beloved matriarch, who'd remained in pain. When the guard arrived in the room, he took one look at the patient and told the nurse that something was very wrong.

"We had just been talking about it in school, how Black and brown people are dying more often in the hospital, and the whole time my grandmother was in the hospital hemorrhaging," Avila said.

Her grandmother lost consciousness and never woke up. The family later learned that an artery had kinked, causing her fatal stroke.

The family was still reeling weeks later when Avila's mother began to complain of headaches and vertigo. Avila conducted a brief neurological exam while visiting and felt certain her mom had a serious problem. A brain scan revealed that her mother had an aneurysm that was too large simply to monitor. Though a surge of Covid-19 delayed the surgery until after Avila's 30th birthday in August, her mother made a full recovery.

* * *

By that fall, all six of the TCU medical students had received Covid boosters, but the shots didn't prevent Avila from becoming sick again, this time a week before she gave birth on Jan. 3, 2022.

She'd enjoyed an easy pregnancy, something she did not take for granted. But the birth "was terrifying," she said. "Everything was going fine until it wasn't."

She and husband Sam arrived that chilly winter morning at Fort Worth's Baylor Scott & White All Saints Medical Center for a scheduled induction at 39 weeks. Avila received an epidural right away and felt no pain, but she was dilating slowly. Her team hooked her up to an intrauterine monitor to make sure the contractions were normal before giving her medicine to accelerate them.

She was shopping on her phone for a pair of boots when a nurse came in to check her progress. When the woman pulled back the sheets, she found Avila in a pool of blood. The nurse rushed to find the doctor as the baby's heartbeat dropped.

"I have seen enough to know how things can go bad really fast," Avila said.

Her obstetrician suggested a cesarean section. Avila agreed to the procedure after learning that she had lost a half-liter of blood in 30 minutes and was dilated only 3 centimeters. She began bleeding faster as they readied her for emergency surgery. A few minutes later, Quentin Samuel Avila emerged pale, struggling to breathe and not crying as much as he should.

"It was the worst feeling ever," Avila said. "I told Sam to go with him and talk to him. He started breathing when he heard Dad's voice."

The nurse took the baby to the neonatal intensive care unit, where his blood sugar stabilized. In the days that followed, Avila rebounded from the C-section with minimal pain as Quentin quickly began to thrive.

Early 2022 was hectic in a far different way for Shah, one of four TCU medical students to enroll in a nine-credit-hour program with the TCU Neeley School of Business. A full-tuition scholarship sealed his decision to take one three-hour evening class a week until February 2023. He finished medical school with a graduate certificate in health policy and management.

"My adviser, Dr. [Ken] Hopper, is a psychiatrist who also has an MBA," Shah said. "We used to have all of these conversations about health care management [and] business, and I know there is theory behind it all, but I was craving a formal education."

To prepare for the Step 1, Shah had moved back in with his parents, who live in McKinney, Texas. He'd leave the house most mornings by 6 to study at

Ive Avila and her husband, Sam, welcomed their first child, Quentin Samuel Avila, in January 2022.

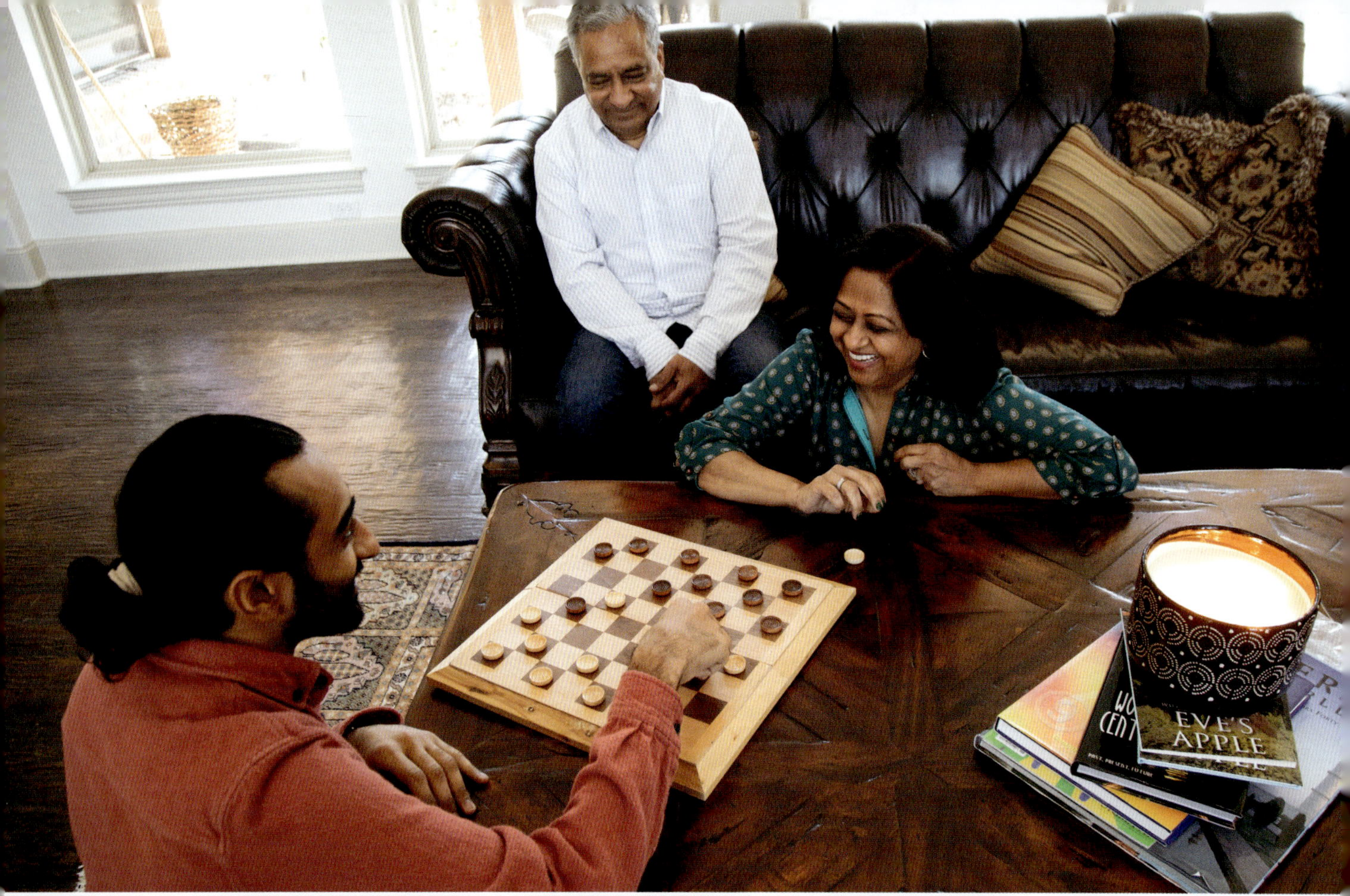
EVE'S APPLE

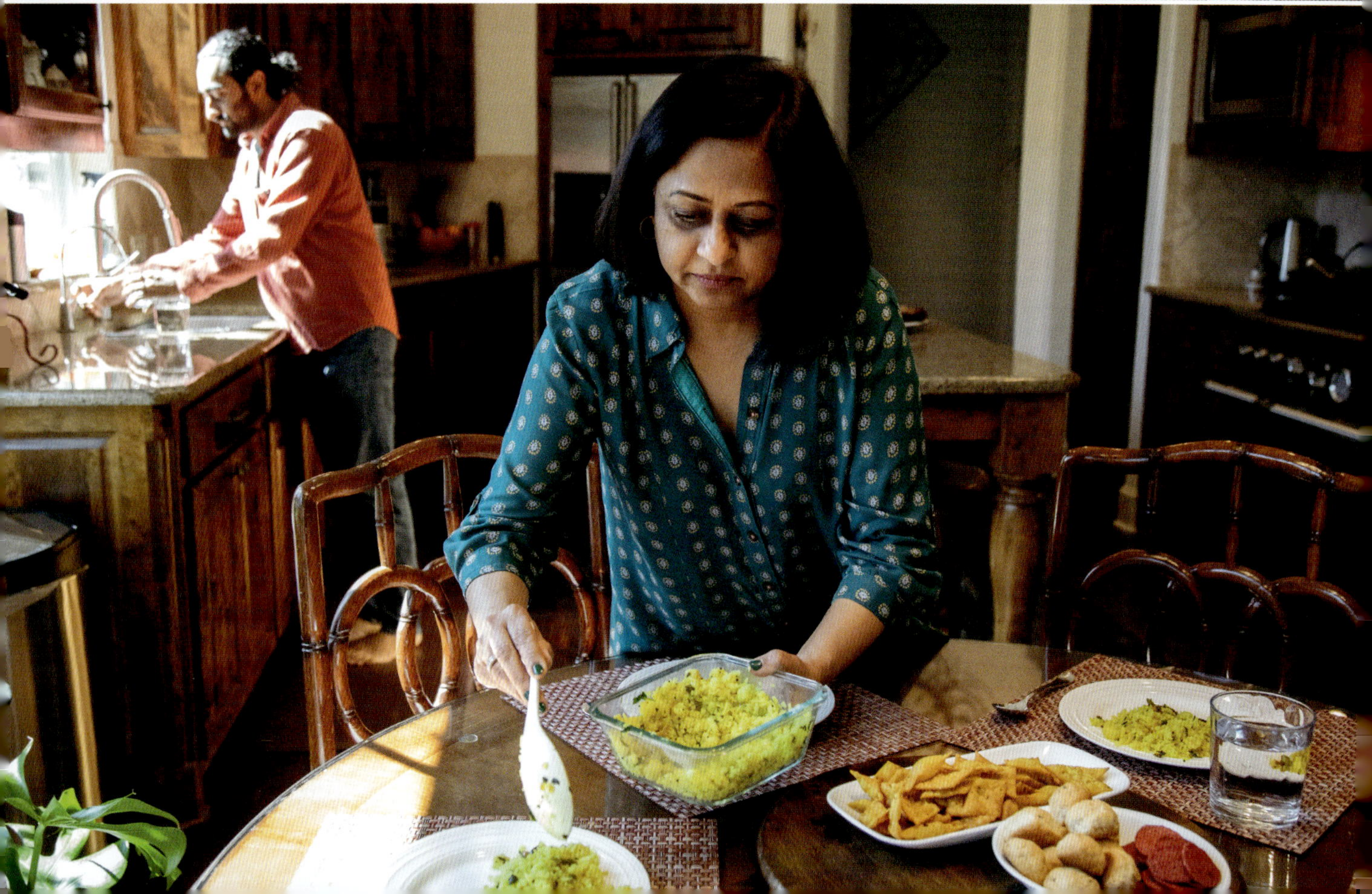

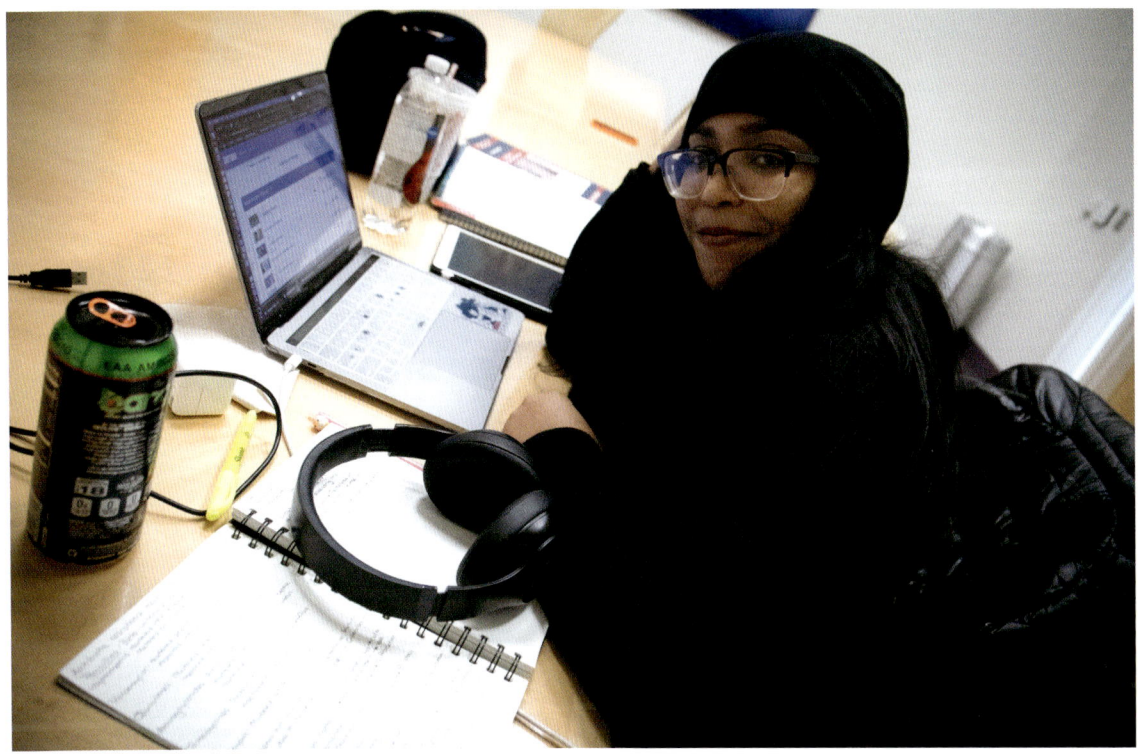

a shared workspace until 7 p.m. After dinner with his mom and dad, he'd hit the books again.

"I'd never seen him work that hard," said his mother, Ila Shah.

Her son had spent the previous year leaning toward otolaryngology. Head and neck surgery is one of the three most competitive specialties in medicine, alongside plastic surgery and dermatology. He needed a strong score.

Shah noticed the toll exam prep was taking on his classmates, so he set up a daily Zoom call where anyone could drop in and study alongside friends. "We were all sharing in the misery," he said. "Studying apart but together seemed to really help."

Kinard and two other third-year students spearheaded an effort to convince the school to allow them more time to prepare. After 48 of her 58 classmates joined the effort, the school gave them until early January to sit for the seven-hour exam.

A school specialist also created individualized study schedules for each student. "I can't begin to describe how much Dr. [Shavonia] Wynn helped me," she said.

In addition to pressure from the Step 1, Kinard said she felt the ongoing strain of dealing with the pandemic. Losefsky described herself as "fatigued with the Covid conversation.

"As soon as someone knows I am in med school, the vaccine comes up," she said. "I feel duty-bound to make it an educational conversation, but it's exhausting."

Particularly when interacting with unvaccinated

Above: Charna Kinard logged hundreds of hours preparing for the Step 1 exam, which all medical students must take before applying to residency programs in the U.S. Left: Shah moved back into the family home advance of his first board exam. His parents, Sunil and Ila Shah, said they were consistently impressed with his work ethic and dedication to medicine.

patients, Kruse felt compelled to fight misinformation. "This is where our school's empathy training has really helped," he said. "It's easy to be compassionate when you are bright-eyed and have had a full night of sleep. They've given us some really useful tools to have tricky conversations no matter the circumstance."

During pediatric rotations in area clinics, Kruse sat in on conversations with teens begging their parents to let them get vaccinated. "Usually kids hate shots," he said, "so that's been a really interesting dynamic to see play out."

* * *

By early 2022, Kruse felt the time had come to decide on a career path.

"I kept telling him that's something no one else can decide for him," his wife, Anabel, said.

Kruse's stellar Step 1 score — plus the equally impressive Step 2 score that he earned later in the spring — put any option in medicine within reach.

Working in a nursing home between college and medical school had given Kruse an awareness of the toll certain specialties can take on both physicians and family members. Many high-achieving medical students gravitate to radiology, ophthalmology, dermatology or anesthesiology. Those specialties have a reputation for offering an appealing lifestyle thanks to the relatively consistent hours. Not coincidentally, those specialties also rank among the most competitive for residencies.

Specialty aside, Kruse had decided early on to work toward the goal of becoming an academic physician, one who can teach and conduct publishable research. In spring 2022, he spoke at a conference in Seattle about his research on the long-term impacts of metformin, a drug used to treat high blood sugar levels caused by Type 2 diabetes.

After months of discussions with physician-

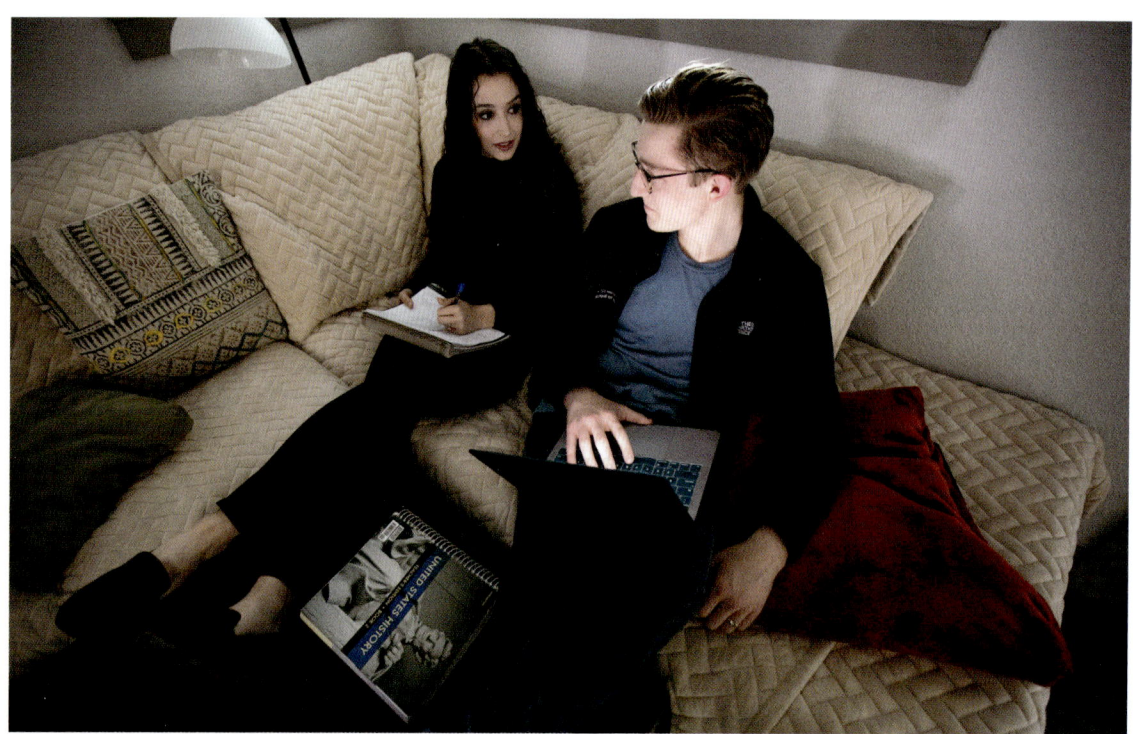

Above: Kruse studied at home alongside his wife, Anabel, who was teaching high school history classes while in Fort Worth. Right: Losefsky, who scrubbed in to surgeries whenever she could, assisted Dr. Joshua Trussell, a general surgeon based in Mansfield, Texas.

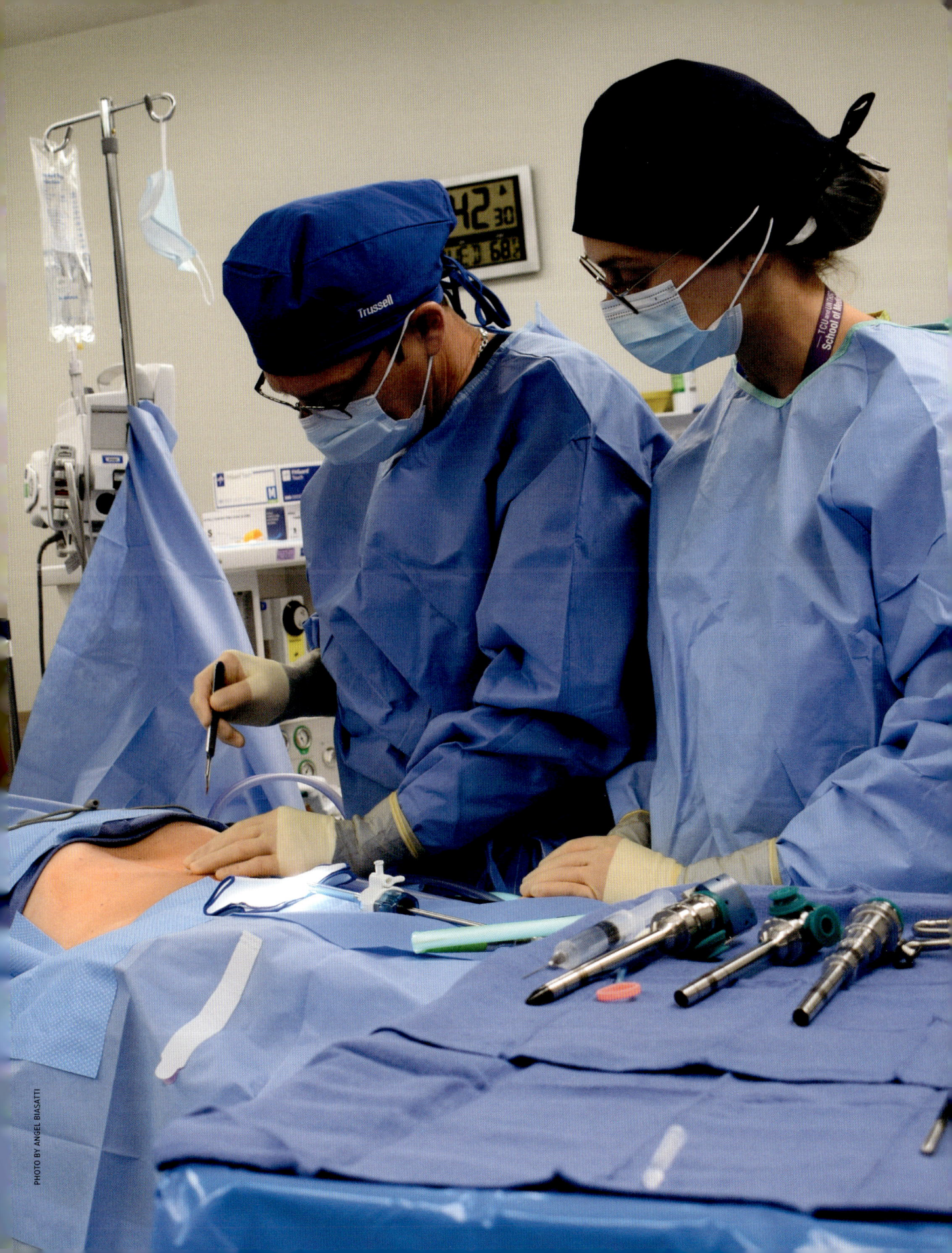

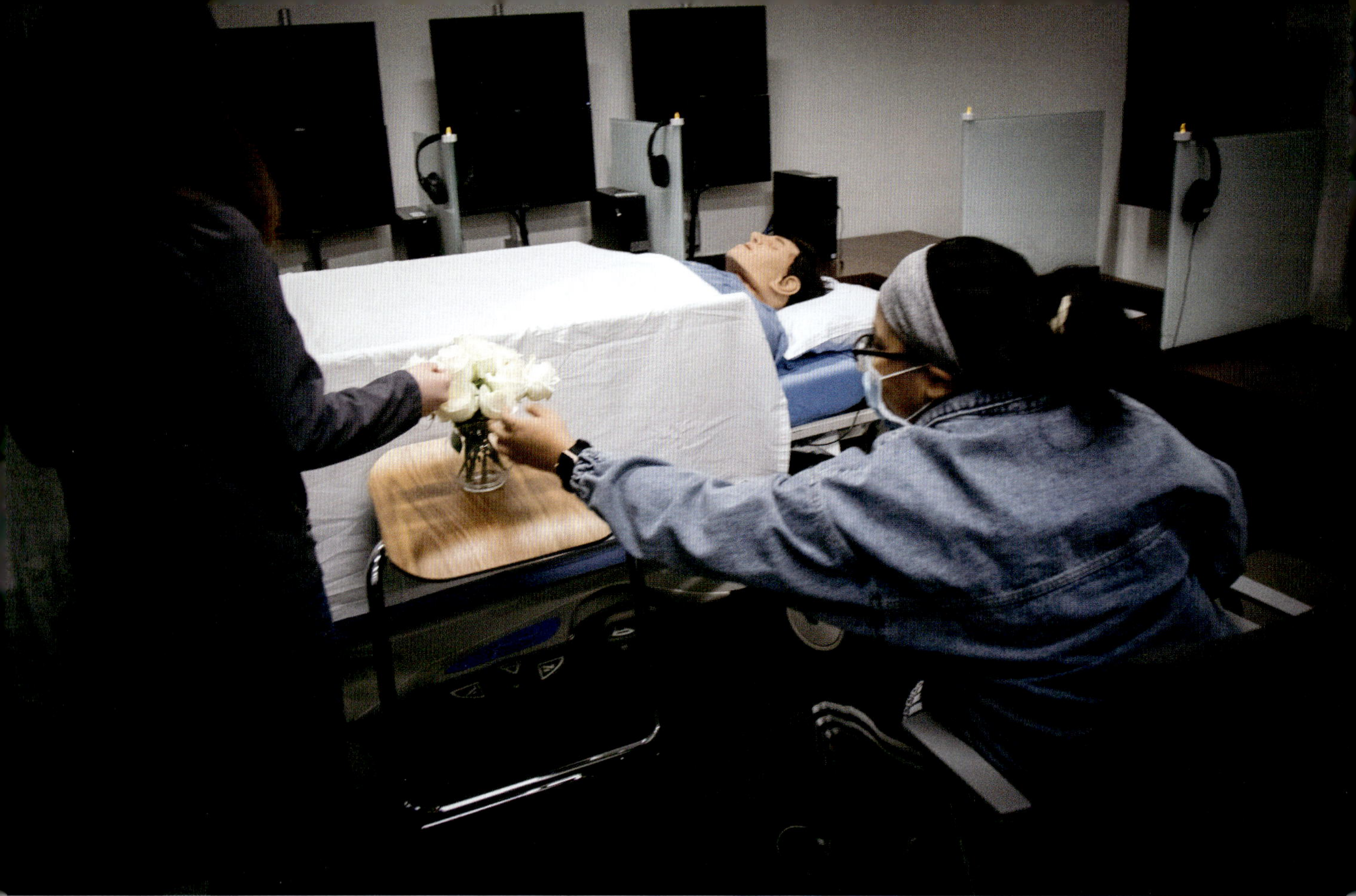

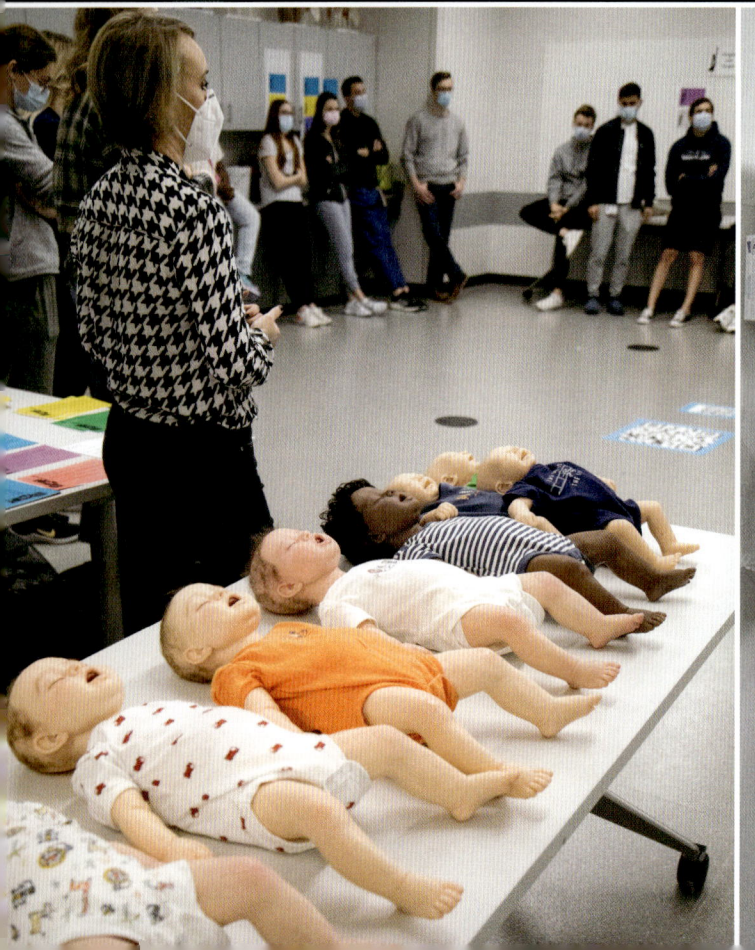
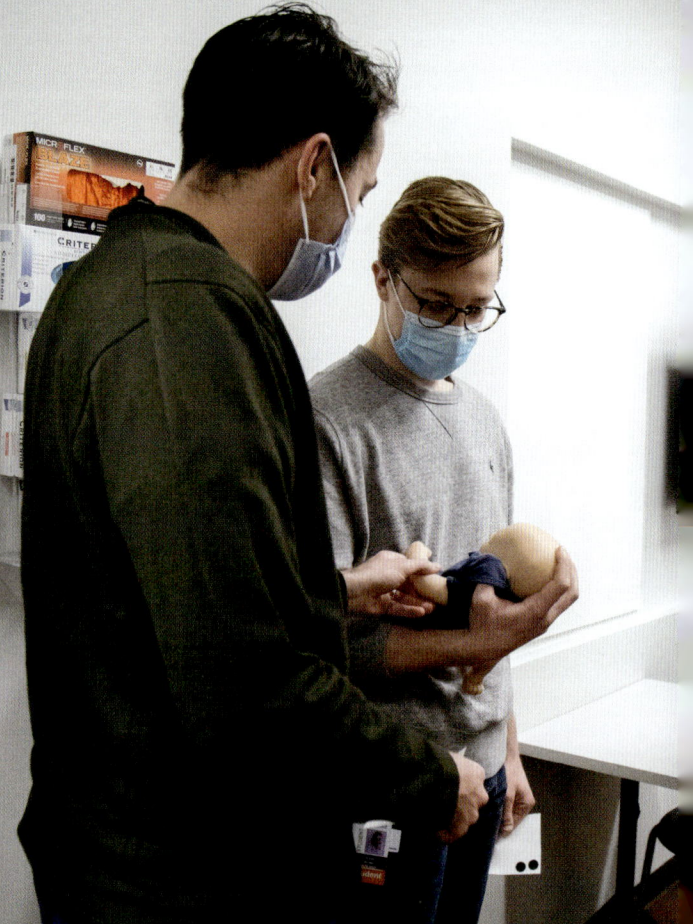

mentors in North Texas and Southern California, along with plenty of soul searching, Kruse chose interventional radiology. Doctors in this specialty treat a host of diseases, cancers included. Among the procedures they perform are needle biopsies, stent placements and angioplasties, which open blocked coronary arteries. Year 1 of the seven-year interventional radiology residency is all surgery.

For his part, Shah agonized over his decision for much of his third year at TCU. While vacillating between head and neck surgery and psychiatry, he kept coming back to the idea that he could make a bigger impact in the arena of mental health.

"I think I can become a good surgeon," he said, "but I can be a great psychiatrist."

So dedicated was Losefsky to becoming a surgeon that she gave her phone number to the surgeons she worked with so they could text her whenever they had an interesting case. Weekly horseback riding lessons helped her stay connected with a lifelong passion, but always, inevitably, she chose to spend time in the operating room when given the opportunity.

Kinard did a rotation at Cook Children's Medical Center in Fort Worth in May 2022, where for the first time she scrubbed in with a Black female surgeon. She'd signed on for that rotation specifically to work with Dr. Kanika Bowen-Jallow, whom she assisted in removing a portion of a dead bowel from a day-old patient.

"These are significant experiences shaping who I will be as a surgeon," said Kinard, who as the Association of American Medical Colleges student representative served as a liaison between TCU and the organization, which seeks to make patient care safe, affordable and equitable.

Avila drew on personal experience when working with OB-GYN patients in various clinical settings.

Avila's husband had driven her to the hospital

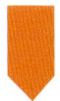

"As a third-year med student, it felt like life was speeding by me. It's sometimes really hard to believe that medical school is almost over."

Quinn Losefsky

in blizzard conditions in winter 2021 as she was miscarrying their first pregnancy. She'd continued her studies without missing a beat and was soon expecting again, but the sorrow of the miscarriage returned those first few weeks of motherhood.

In the days after her son's birth, Avila "couldn't even look at his baby blankets, his bottle or pacifier without feeling this intense panic. I do remember thinking, 'Here I am holding this baby, and there's another baby I should be holding, and I'll never get that opportunity.'

"I've seen patients come in with postpartum depression, but I think a lot more women get it and don't talk about it," Avila said. "Why doesn't this get talked about?"

She rejoined the class online a few weeks after her son's arrival and kept up with her assignments while taking six weeks off from clinical rotation. It was an exhausting time.

"There is something to be said about allowing a mother and child to have that time uninterrupted," she said. "I really think we have a lot of work to do in giving medical professionals the time they need with their babies."

* * *

Clockwise from top: Students including Miki Edwards, left, and Kinard participated in an extended exercise about domestic violence as part of their classroom training. Part of the role-playing included a mock funeral; Tom Roser, left, and Kruse held a "baby" as part of the training; The Burnett School of Medicine uses baby-sized manikins to teach students about caring for infants.

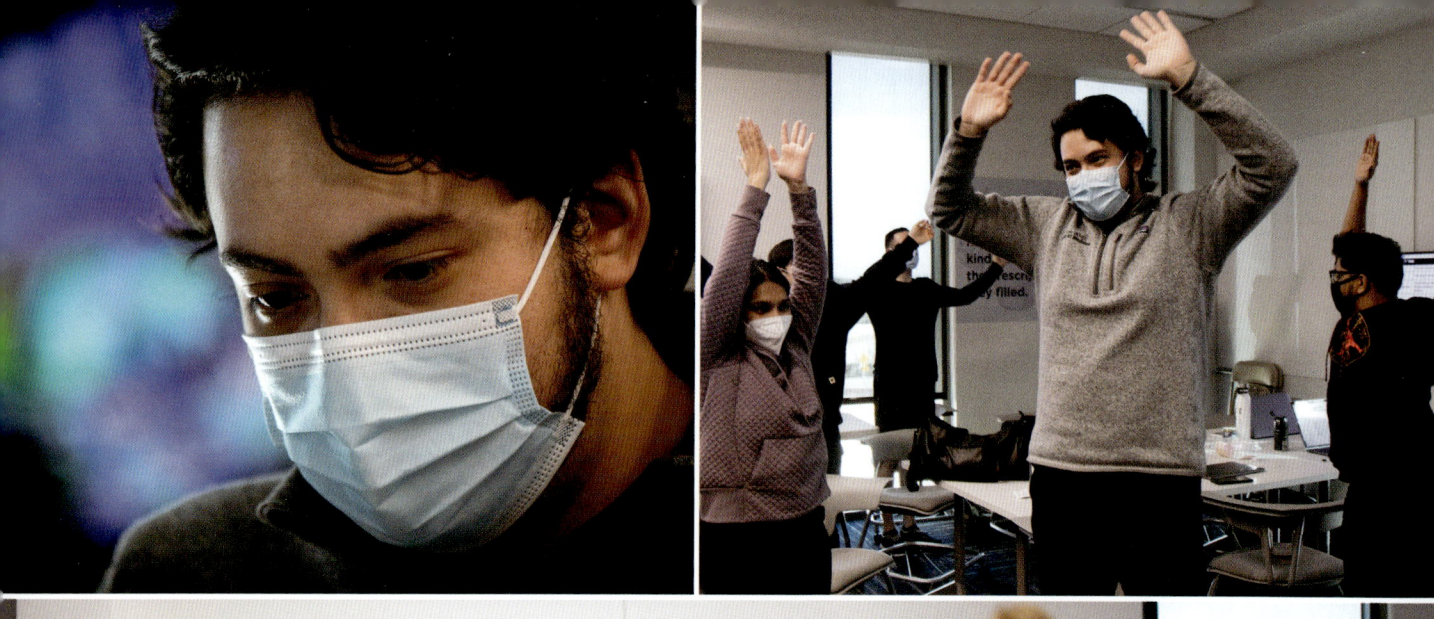

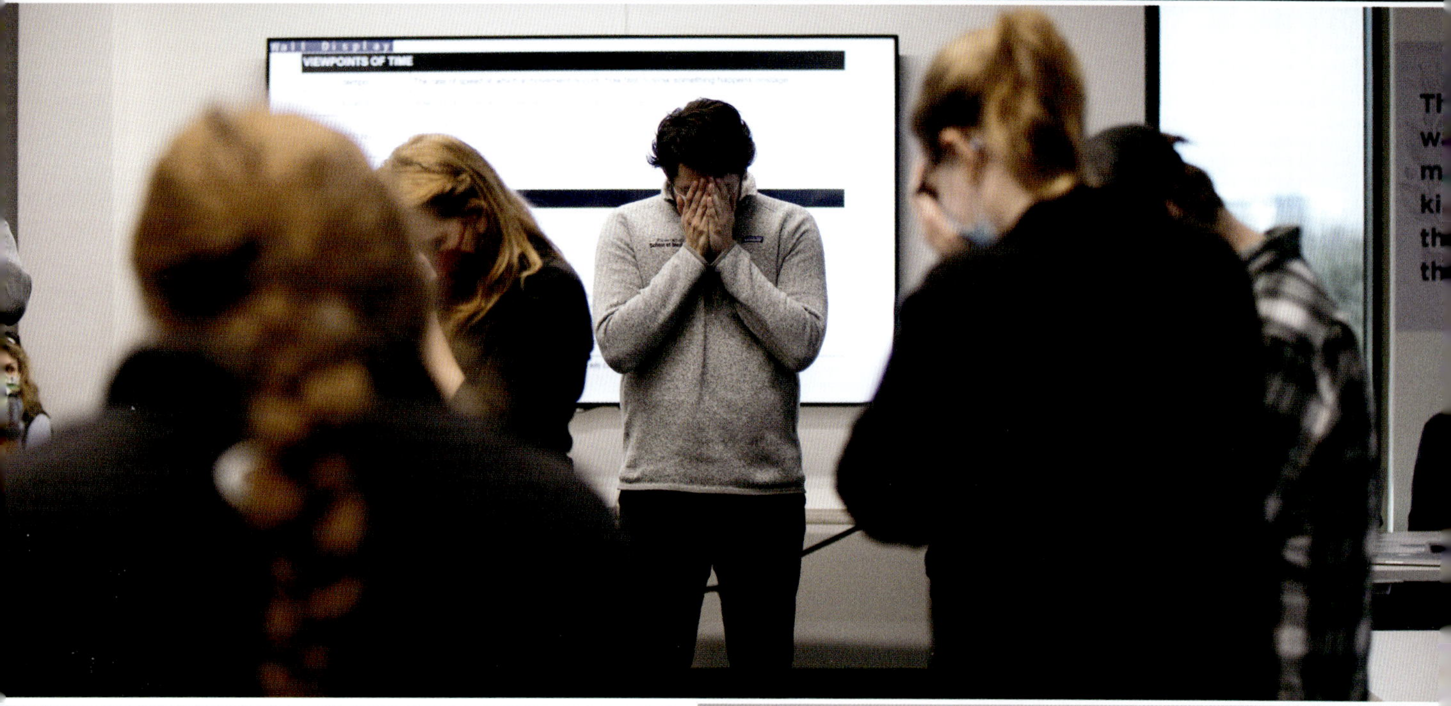

Empathy and compassion are woven into all aspects of the Anne Burnett Marion School of Medicine curriculum. In their third year, students engage in various training sessions to enhance their ability to relate to others, particularly their patients.

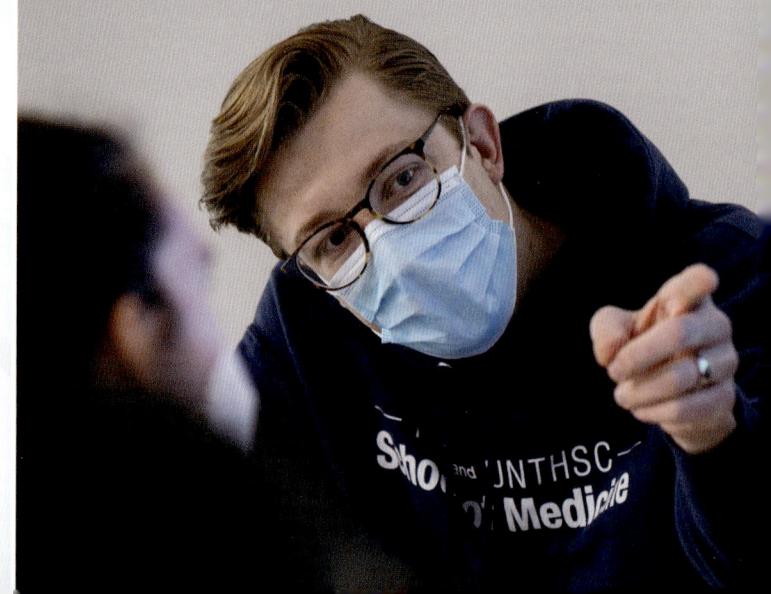

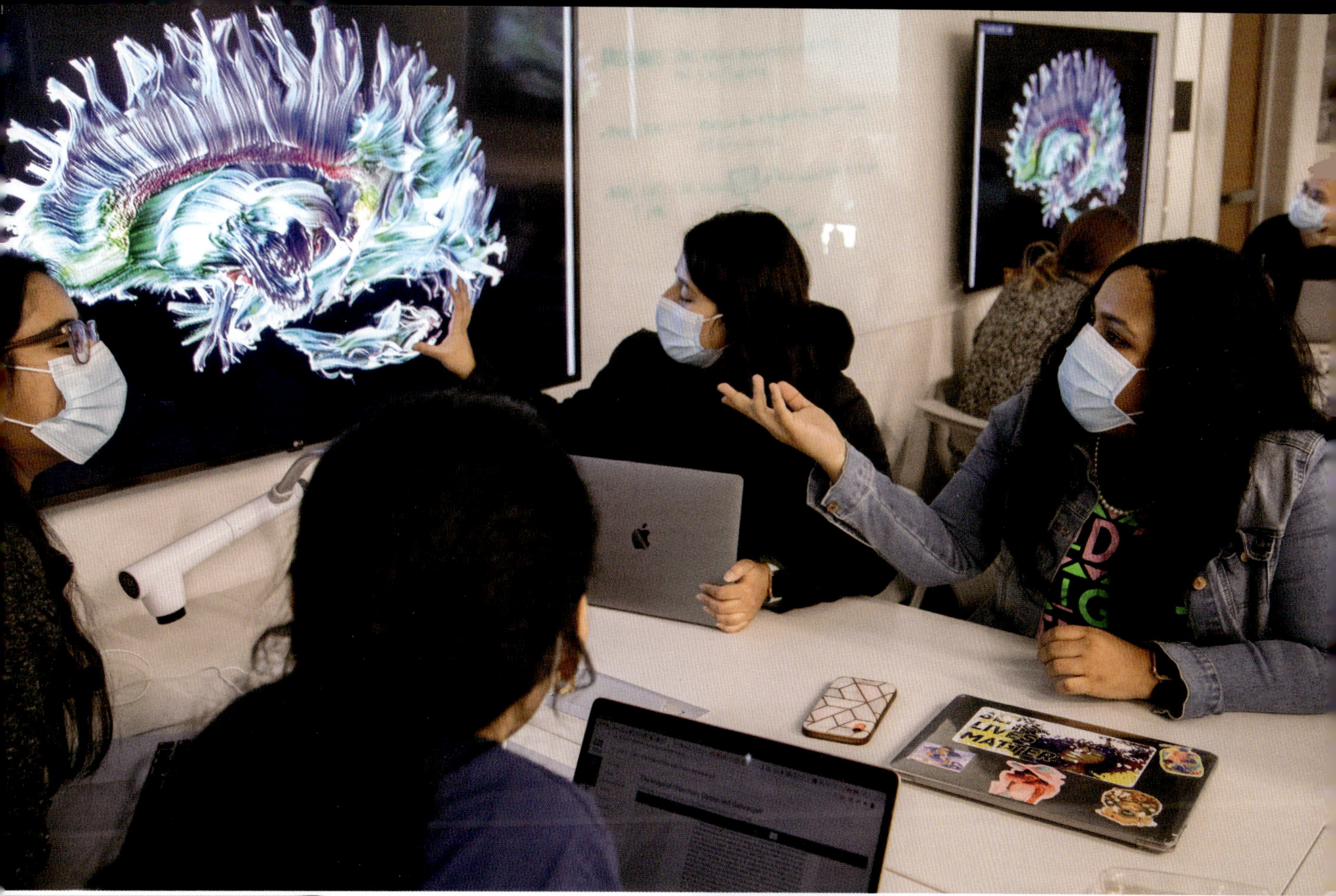

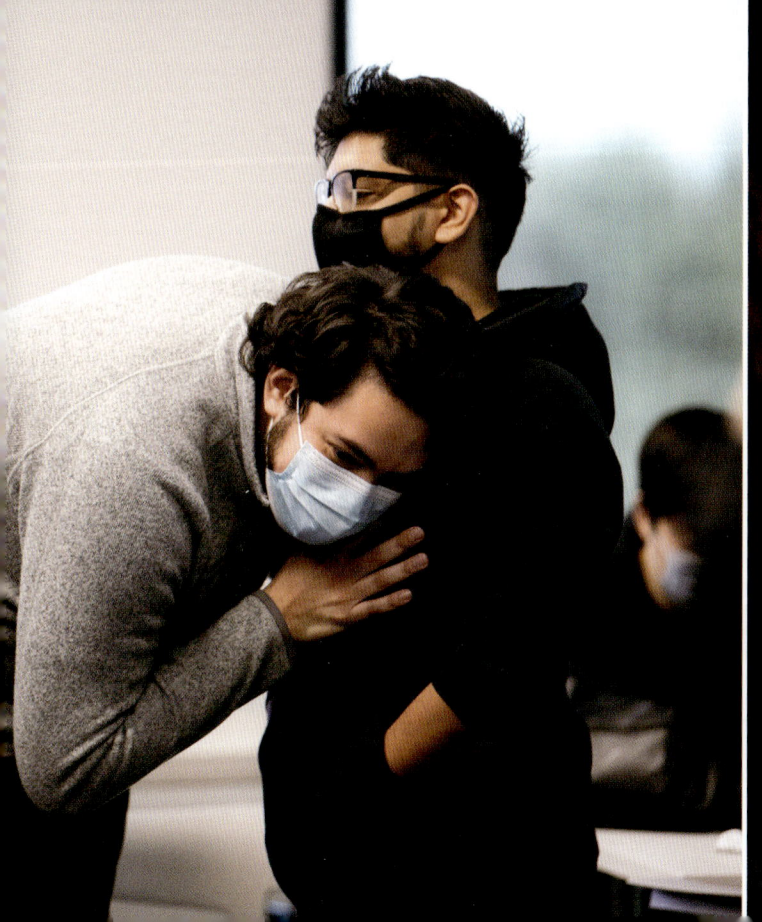
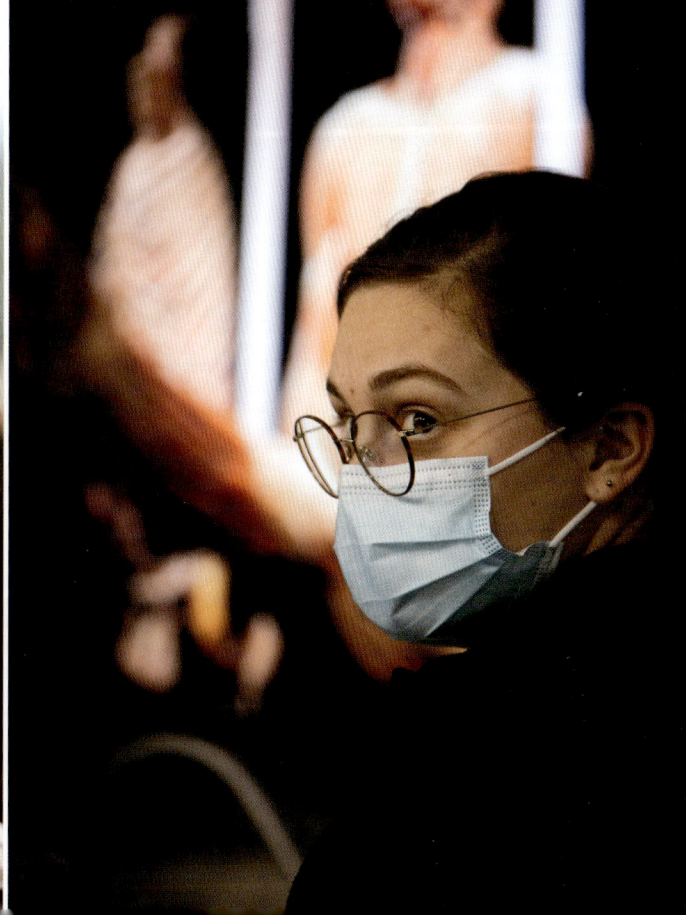

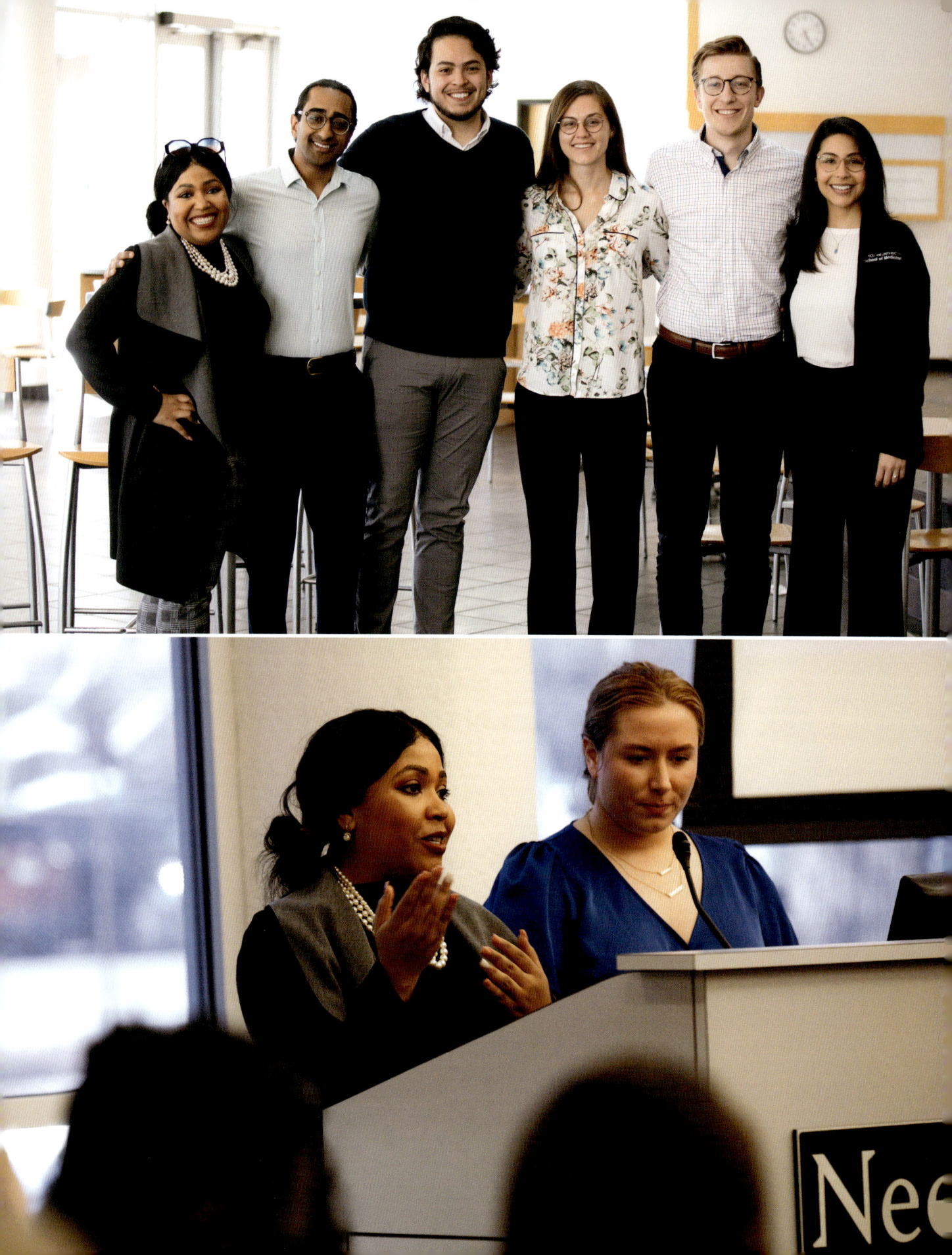

Esparza, who took the Step 2 exam in late June 2022, had something to smile about when he was named an ElevateMeD Scholar, a program for physician leaders from historically underrepresented racial and ethnic groups. In addition to a $10,000 scholarship, the award came with ongoing mentoring and financial-planning education. Like Kinard and Kruse, he aspired to work at a medical school one day.

In April 2022, Shah traveled to Washington, D.C., to speak about his research at a conference on psychiatry. Deepening crises in the U.S., including skyrocketing rates of teen depression and substance use, convinced him to focus on mental health. He also credited his experience at the Neeley School of Business with helping him reflect on the motivations and rewards of a career as a physician.

"I know my intentions for entering medicine are altruistic at their core, but somewhere over the last grueling year I have shifted to a more cynical mindset that wants acknowledgment for my acumen and retribution for the hundreds of thousands of dollars I am spending on my medical education," he wrote in a paper for one of his business classes, Health Care in the U.S.

Shah said the Neeley classes helped remind him of his true purpose in pursuing a medical degree. "No matter what specialty," he said, "I am absolutely dedicated to giving my patients the very best care."

"This hasn't been an easy journey," Flynn said toward the end of the third year for the Class of 2023. "They are the trailblazers for our school, and we are indebted to these young people who have put confidence in us."

With Year 3 behind them, the students would never again come together for formal medical training. Nor would they take any more tests administered by the Burnett School of Medicine. The academic part of

"This hasn't been an easy journey. They are the trailblazers for our school, and we are indebted to these young people who have put confidence in us."

Dr. Stuart D. Flynn

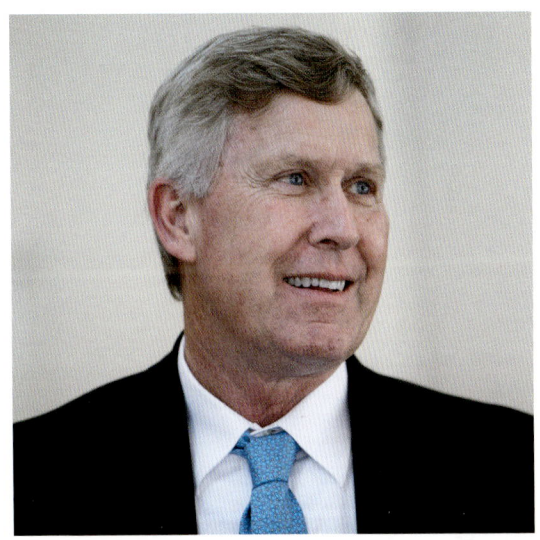

Dr. Stuart D. Flynn, is the founding dean of the Anne Burnett Marion School of Medicine.

medical school was over for TCU's inaugural cohort of medical students.

"As a third-year med student, it felt like life was speeding by me," Losefsky said with a year to go before collecting her second diploma from TCU.

"It's sometimes really hard to believe that medical school is almost over." ✦

Opposite page, top: The *TCU Magazine* six joined their classmates for a presentation of community projects in March 2022. Bottom: Kinard and Sam Evans presented their project results on breaking down health care barriers.

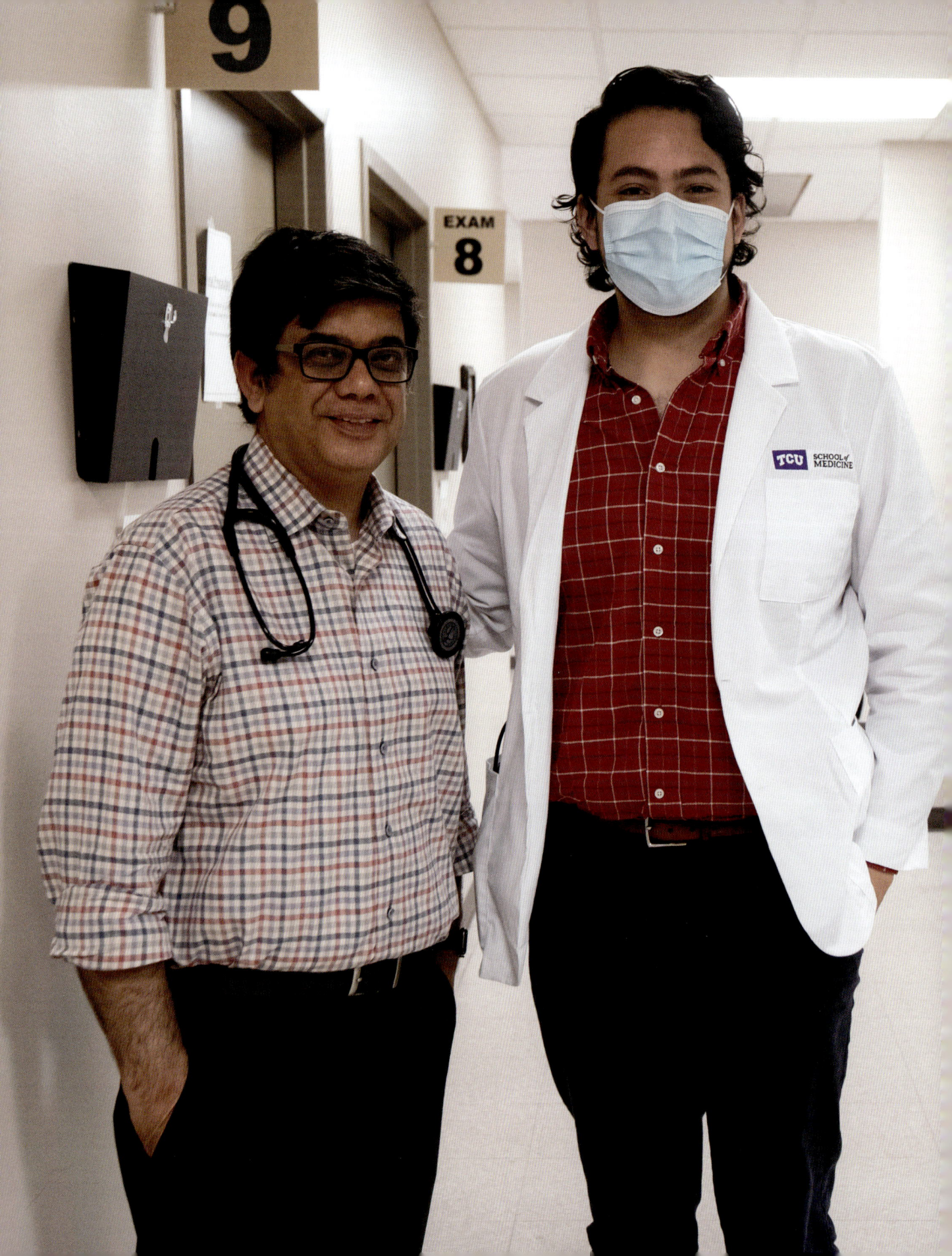

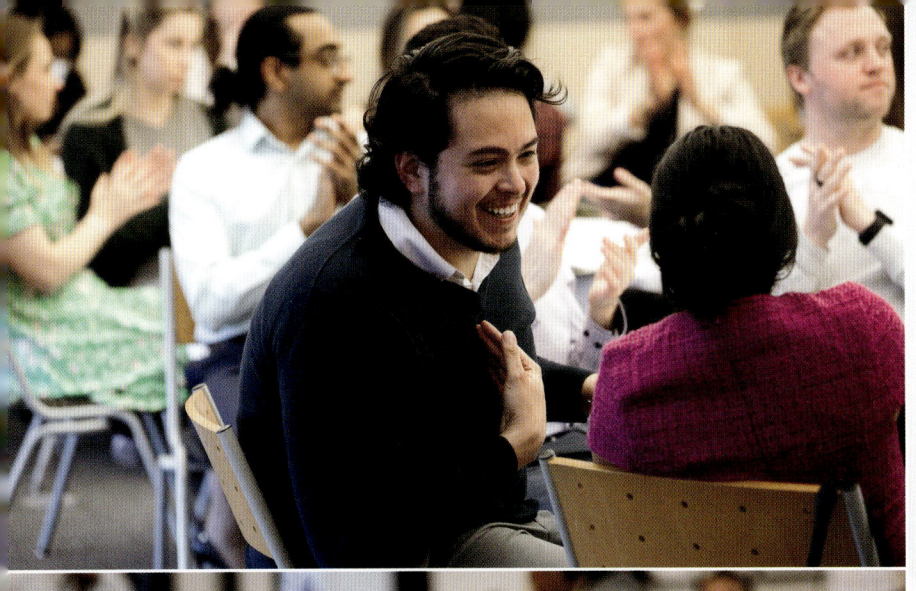

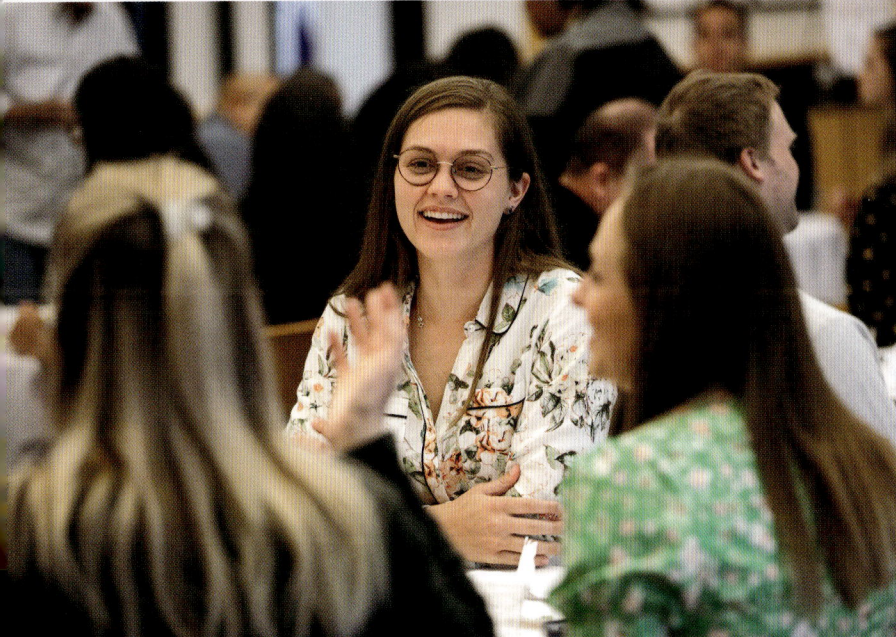

Opposite page: Esparza credited
Dr. Sumeesh Dhawan, who specializes
in internal medicine, for being a
transformational mentor in his
educational journey.

This page: Burnett School of Medicine
students celebrated and shared the
results of their many community projects
during presentations at the TCU Neeley
School of Business.

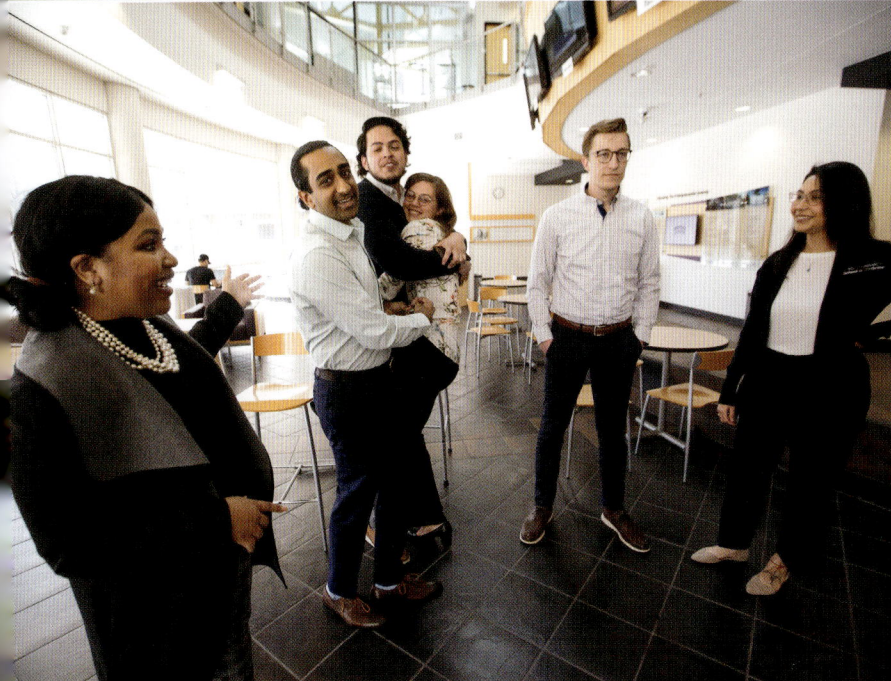

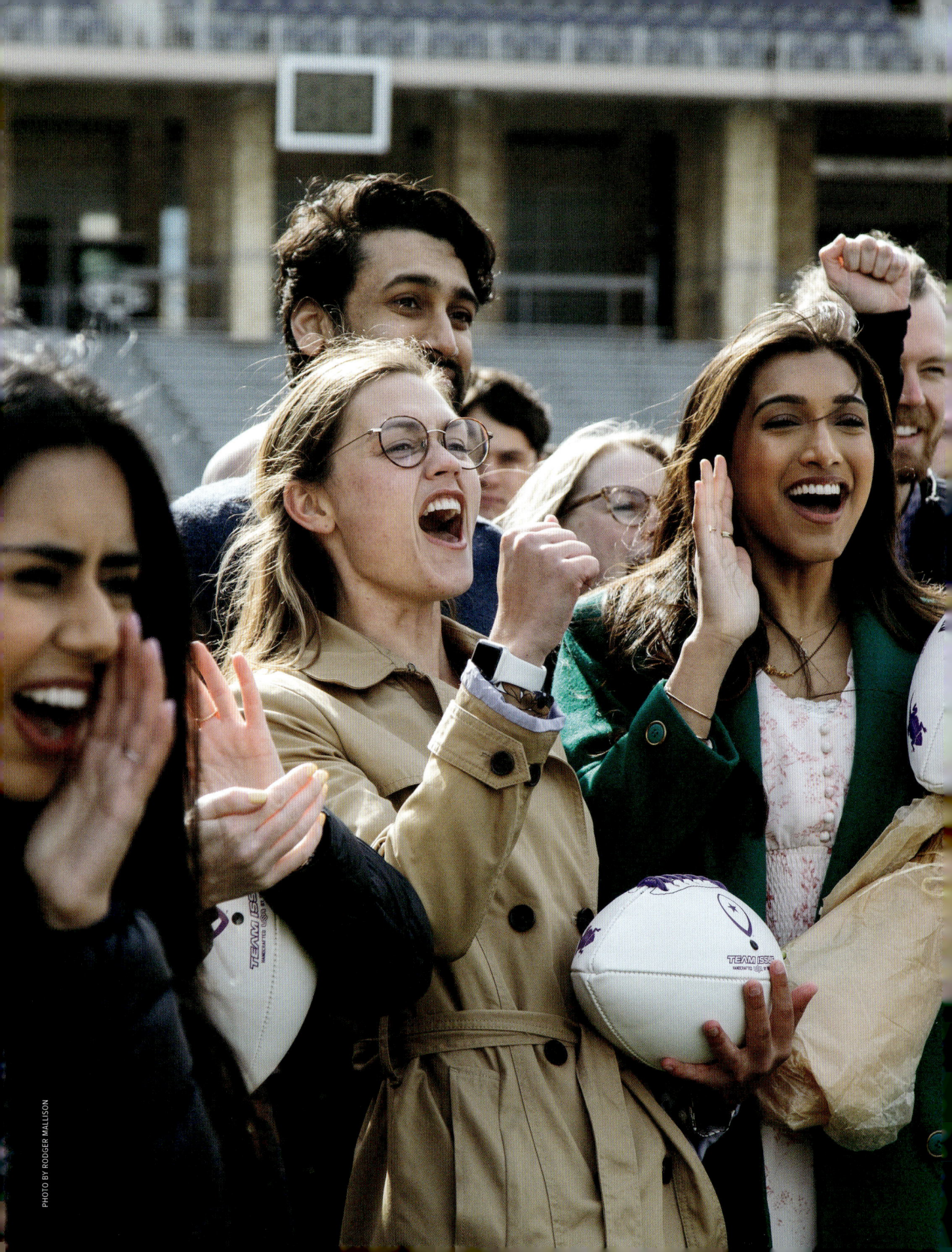

YEAR FOUR

2022-23

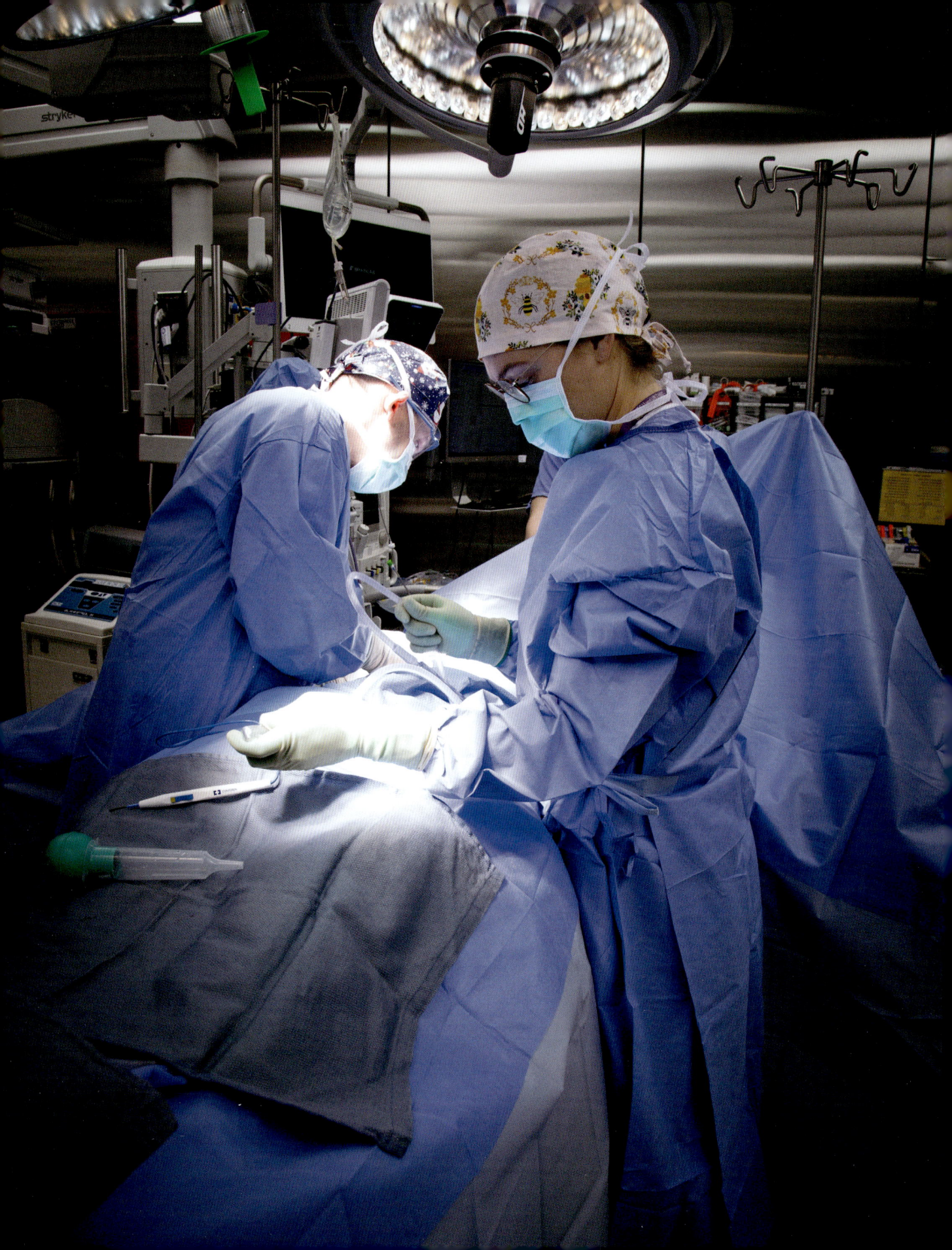

The Class of 2023

Economic issues and the addiction crisis dominated headlines during the final year of medical school for the Class of 2023.

High rates of inflation and labor shortages weakened the economy. The 12-month period ending in January 2023 also saw the opioid crisis claim a record 109,000 lives in the U.S., most of which were blamed on fentanyl, a potent synthetic drug.

The Anne Burnett Marion School of Medicine reached its capacity upon welcoming its fourth class of students in July 2022. The Class of 2026 was 62 percent women and 38 percent men, with an average MCAT score of 509 and an overall grade point average of 3.66.

Five of the incoming medical students were TCU graduates, with 11 Texas residents in the class. Twenty-eight percent entered the school with graduate degrees in everything from global health and film production to nutrition and biomolecular science.

"We now have a full campus of 240 medical students who have chosen a new approach to medical education as their calling," Dean Stuart D. Flynn said at the start of the medical school's fourth year. "These students will have a unique viewpoint on the role that empathetic communication plays in better patient care. That is how we help patients get better health outcomes and improve community health overall."

As TCU celebrated its sesquicentennial, the university hit a milestone when its first class of doctors graduated in May 2023. The new MDs embarked on residencies in specialties including general surgery, internal medicine, anesthesiology, psychiatry, emergency medicine, family medicine, obstetrics-gynecology, pediatrics and orthopedic surgery.

* * *

Jonas Kruse's final year of medical school began with a full-circle moment as he stood at a podium inside Amon G. Carter Stadium to welcome the 60 newest medical students to the Burnett School of Medicine. In his speech at the white coat ceremony in July 2022, he told the Class of 2026 how he had begun to see patients days into his first year at TCU.

Such immediate patient interaction helps set the university apart from all but a handful of the more than 150 schools granting MD degrees in the U.S. Kruse and his classmates spent a total of 84 weeks doing clinical rotations during their first three years.

"As a triumphant fourth-year medical student with thousands of clinical hours under my belt, I still don't have all the answers," Kruse told the crowd. "What I've come to learn is that the residents I'm working with, the fellows I'm working with and even the attendings also don't have all of the answers."

Nine months later, Kruse and his 51 graduating classmates learned the answer to the biggest question about how their careers would take shape when they found out where they would be heading for residency.

For the Class of 2023, the medical school experience proved exhilarating and discouraging, thrilling and tedious. For the fourth-year students on the verge of becoming medical doctors, the focus on their futures at times felt overwhelming.

"It's hard not to go down a rabbit hole thinking about residency," Quinn Losefsky said.

Quinn Losefsky assisted Dr. Elliot Waters in removing a chemotherapy port at Texas Health Harris Methodist Hospital Fort Worth.

"There were points when it seemed like all I did was worry about residency," Edmundo Esparza said.

"Residency," Kruse said, "was always on my mind."

From the moment the students matriculated at TCU's medical school, they began to feel anxious about the milestones that would determine the course of their careers. Would they do well on the medical licensing exams? Once they received their results from the Step 1 and the Step 2, the students had to choose a specialty that fit their interests, talents and lifestyle expectations.

To practice medicine as licensed physicians in the U.S., doctors first complete a residency lasting from three to seven years. TCU's inaugural class of medical students were now deciding between university-based residency programs and community programs focusing on patient care.

Decisions, decisions.

To prepare the students for residency, the final year of medical school centers on hospital rotations, called away rotations, at home and around the country. The fourth-years were never all in the same city at the same time until convening in Fort Worth for Match Week in March 2023, when residency placements were announced.

These away rotations typically last a month, with students focusing on a specific discipline, anything from radiology to urology.

TCU's medical students are permitted to pursue as many as four away rotations, which serve as an audition of sorts for residency placement. The school encourages students to spend a month at hospitals outside of Tarrant County to expand their educational horizons and possibly gain letters of recommendation. Many gravitate to aways at programs that top their application lists.

"Dean Flynn told us to explore as much as possible," Kruse said. "On aways, you learn the resident culture and see what opportunities exist for residents to be involved in research as well as getting to know faculty members."

"If you know the discipline you want to go into and you think you know where you'd like to do this training, it's very helpful to do an elective rotation there," Flynn said. "It's used more strategically than when I was a student, but it's really valuable to see other perspectives, even to see the same diagnosis but how they address it from different angles and perspectives."

* * *

Losefsky was the first in her class to venture beyond North Texas. She spent May 2022 in Brooklyn, New York, working at a hospital affiliated with Cornell University. The difference in expectations and levels of autonomy for residents on the East

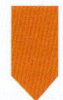

"As a triumphant fourth-year medical student with thousands of clinical hours under my belt, I still don't have all the answers. What I've come to learn is that the residents I'm working with, the fellows I'm working with and even the attendings also don't have all of the answers."

Jonas Kruse

Jonas Kruse traveled the country exploring options for residency programs during his fourth year of medical school at TCU.

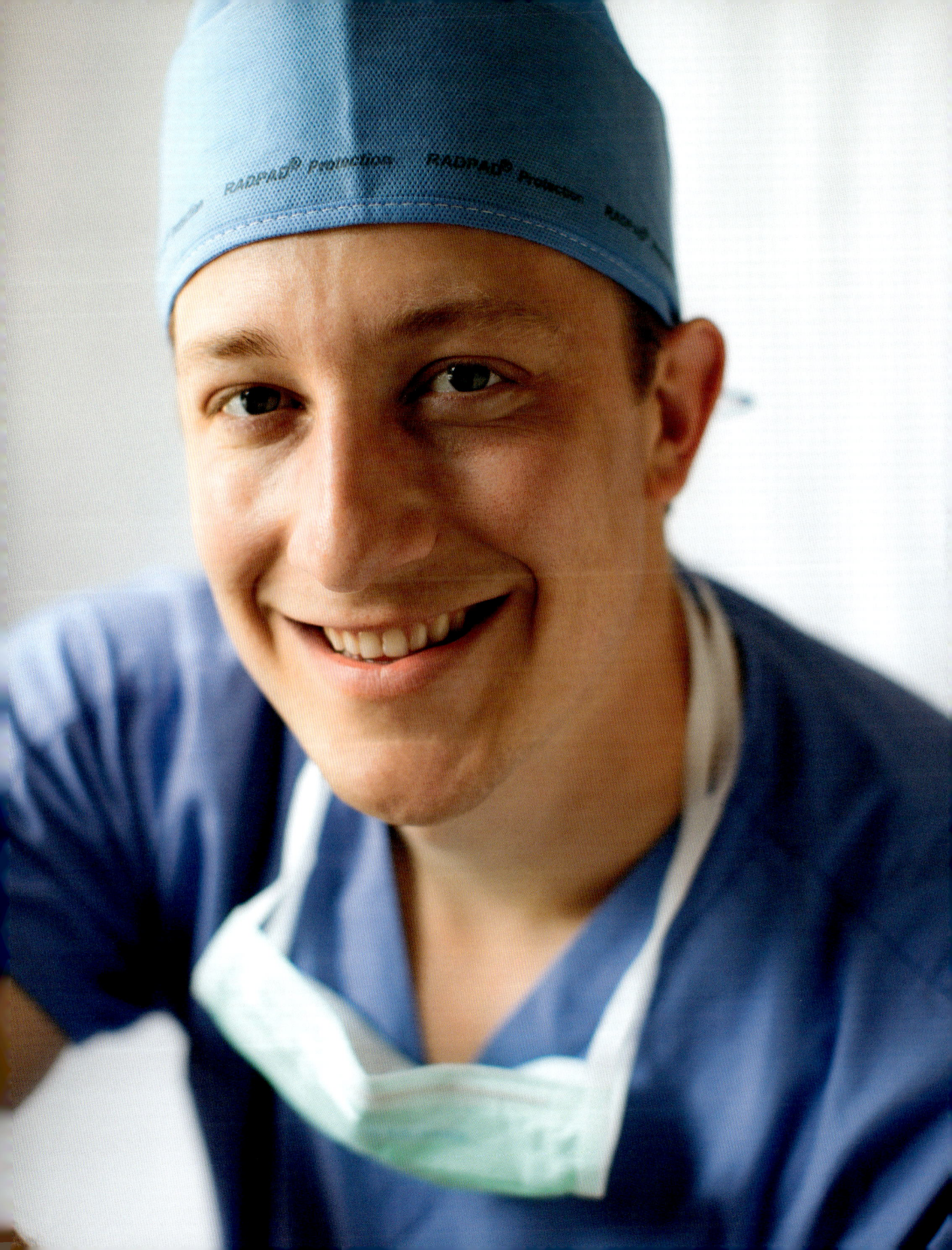

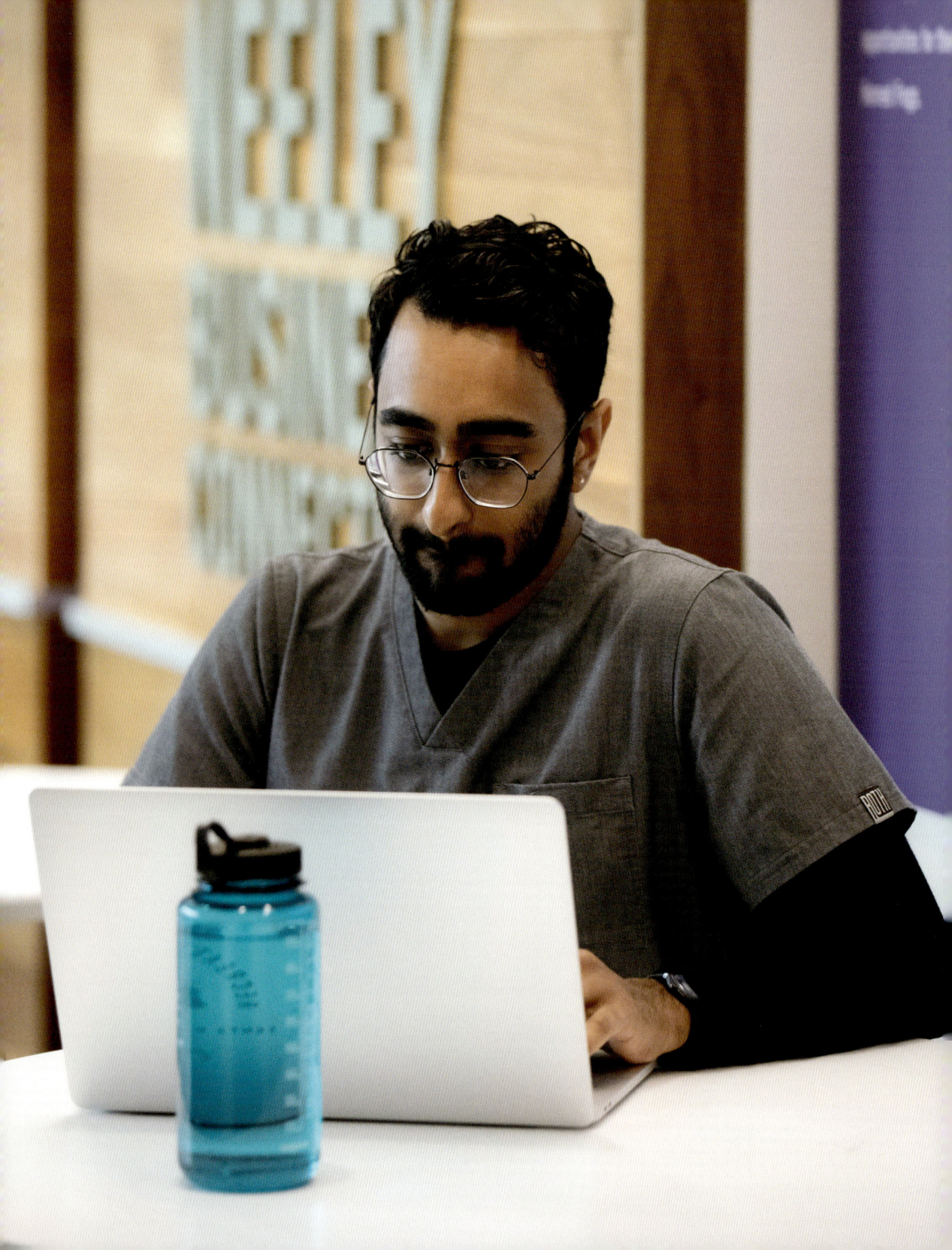

Coast surprised her. When a surgeon let her peel a gallbladder from a liver, a third-year resident told her he'd never seen a medical student do that before.

More than once, Losefsky caught the staff at New York-Presbyterian Brooklyn Methodist Hospital off guard by showing up on her day off, asking to help. She wanted to squeeze every moment of learning from her away rotation, one of two she did in a span of four months.

Losefsky worked at the burn unit at the University of California, San Diego in August 2022. Operating rooms there are kept at a sweltering 90 degrees to prevent hypothermia in burn patients, whose injuries often mean they can no longer thermoregulate.

She bought moisture-wicking undershirts and prepared for extra discomfort while operating, which can be physically demanding under ideal circumstances. She'd learned early on that hunger, thirst, tense muscles, stiff necks and tired feet come with the territory for most surgical specialties.

Losefsky marveled at the intensity and focus most surgeons maintained, particularly when something went wrong. She also admired people skilled at overseeing teams that included an anesthesiologist, nurses and scrub technicians. "The surgeon is really the quarterback," she said. "When the surgeon is not only good at cutting but also at leading others, the outcomes can be so much better for the patient."

Ultimately, she didn't pursue burn work, largely because the procedures felt less exciting and invigorating to her than those she'd encountered in general surgery. She savored the sheer variety of cases that most general surgeons undertake.

Midway through his third year of medical school, Kruse watched an interventional radiologist remove blood clots from the brain of a stroke patient who regained the ability to speak 10 minutes later.

"It was a light-bulb moment for me," said Kruse, who went on to co-author three chapters in an interventional radiology research textbook and join a research team from Stanford University that

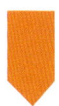

"If you know the discipline you want to go into and you think you know where you'd like to do this training, it's very helpful to do an elective rotation there. ... It's really valuable to see other perspectives, even to see the same diagnosis but how they address it from different angles and perspectives."

Dr. Stuart D. Flynn

presented study findings in Barcelona, Spain. He also founded TCU's vascular interventional radiology and neurology interest groups and helped create a case competition at the annual Academic Interventional Radiology Symposium.

Despite the added expense of aways — travel and housing mostly — Kruse did rotations in interventional radiology at Mount Sinai in New York City, Vanderbilt University in Nashville, UCLA and Kaiser Permanente, also in Los Angeles. Each ranks among the most prestigious programs in the country.

He relished his time in out-of-state hospitals despite having to leave his wife, who taught high school history, at home in Fort Worth with the couple's rescue boxers, Harley and Hank. "Part of what motivated me to work so hard was knowing that Anabel was making a sacrifice for me, too, and that I didn't want to waste a single moment of these opportunities," Kruse said.

"I think I scared the third-years when I told their class that away rotations are not a vacation," he said.

Dilan Shah prepared for a class at the TCU Neeley School of Business. He was one of several medical students awarded a scholarship to pursue a health care management program alongside his medical degree.

"You should be the first one in in the mornings and the last one out. You have everything on the line when you're at an away."

During the second half of medical school, Esparza flirted with pursuing a specialty in pathology before deciding on internal medicine. He liked the idea of seeing patients only in a hospital, he said, and "in internal medicine, I don't have to choose an exact path right away."

He also gravitated toward working with immigrant, underserved and uninsured communities. "Those populations have a different view on medicine," he said. "They know you're on their side and that you want to help."

Financial constraints meant Esparza did only one away rotation, at the University of California,

San Diego. The extreme professionalism of the staff impressed him.

Shah spent January 2023 shadowing Mike Sanborn, then president and CEO of Baylor Scott & White All Saints Medical Center - Fort Worth. "There are so many things going on behind the scenes in the system and in the city," Shah said. "His job is working on 60 projects all at once. You're constantly doing something different."

Between Thanksgiving and Christmas, Shah did an away rotation at Harbor-UCLA Medical Center, a joint venture between the university and Los Angeles County. He worked with a diverse patient population, many of whom had been brought to the county hospital by law enforcement.

"You see things there that you only read about,"

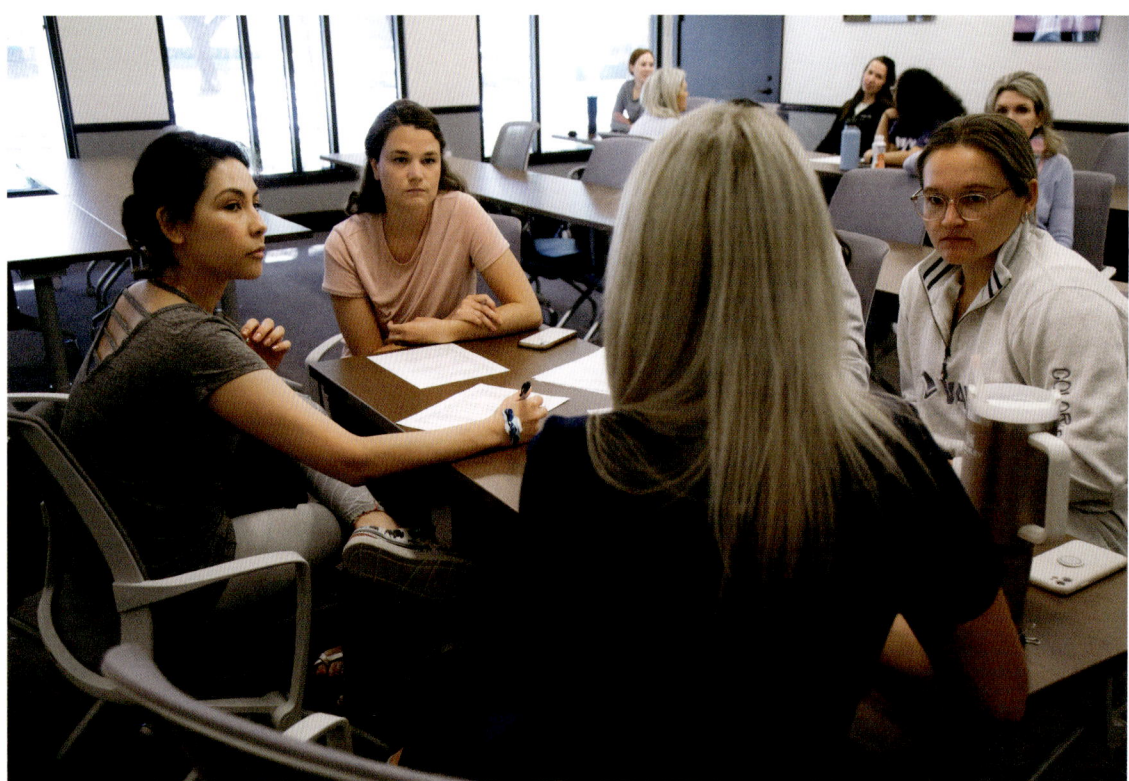

Above: Weeks before graduation, the fourth-year medical students attended a transition-to-residency class. Future OB-GYNs Ive Avila, left, Kathryn Biddle and Shelby Wildish listened to Dr. Adrianne Deem, who practices in Fort Worth. Right: Charna Kinard aimed to return to the Midwest for her residency program.

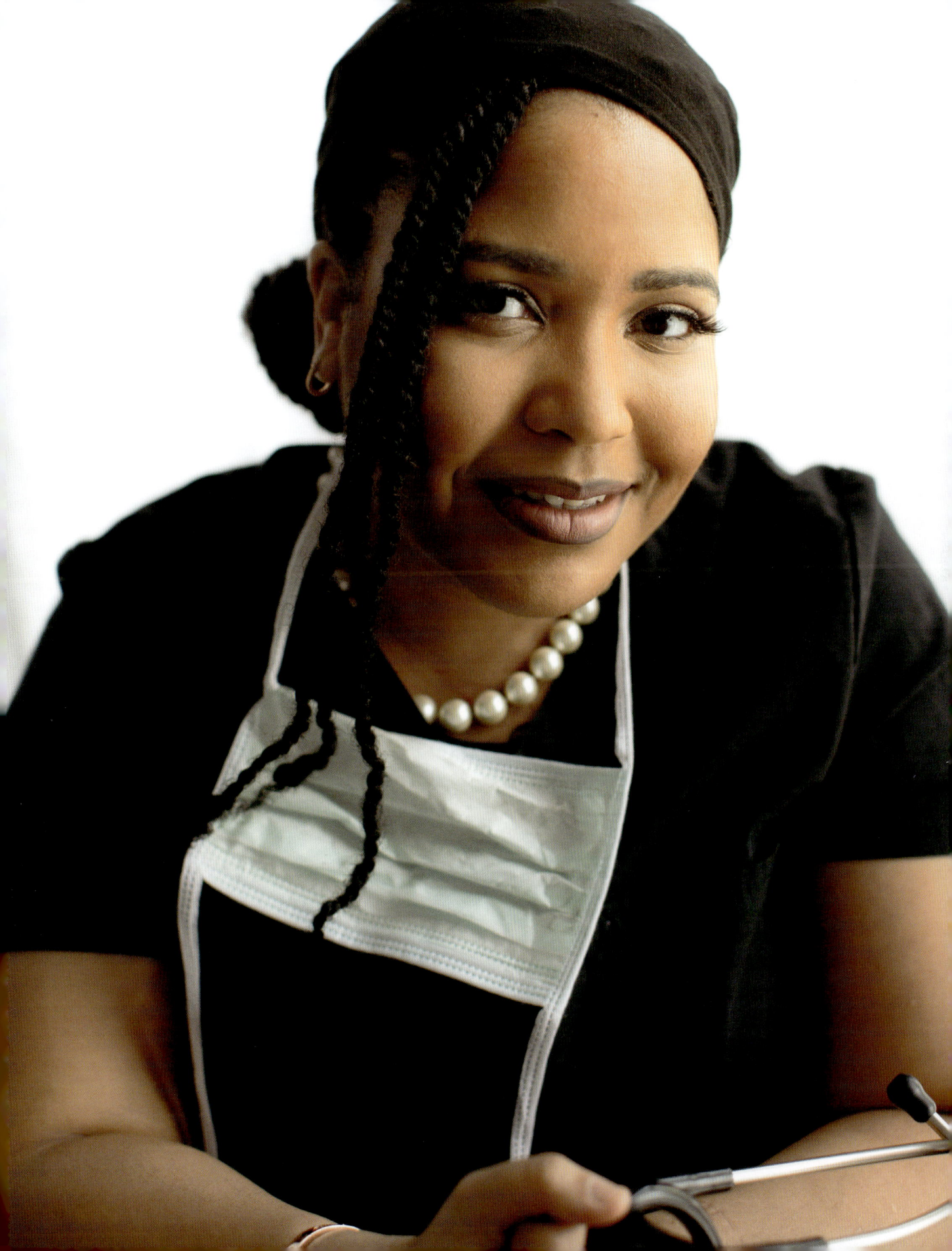

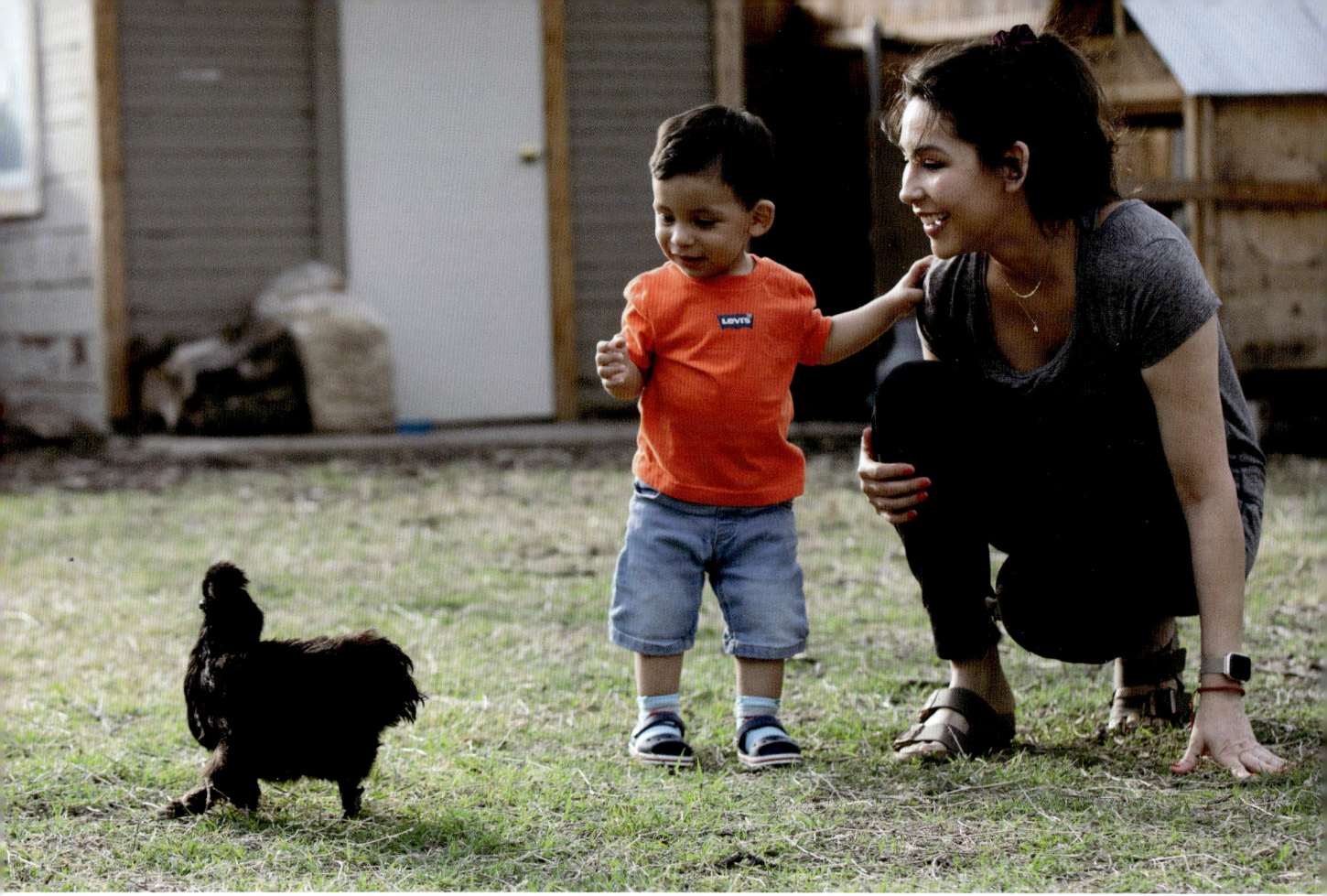

Avila and her son, Quentin, enjoyed a moment with Licorice, one of the family's pet chickens.

Shah said, noting how people from all over the world fly to L.A. in search of Hollywood dreams while in the throes of manic episodes. One patient experiencing such an episode drove a car off the side of a highway to see what would happen. Shah helped manage the man's psychiatric medications while he recovered from extensive physical injuries.

In the final months of 2021, Charna Kinard did back-to-back away rotations in surgery at the Mayo Clinic in Rochester, Minnesota, and the University of Chicago. "There's nothing like being completely immersed in a surgery where everyone is working toward one goal," she said, "helping the patient on the table."

Ive Avila never wavered from wanting to deliver babies and work with women on issues related to sexual and reproductive health.

After welcoming their son, Quentin, midway through her third year of medical school, Avila and her husband decided to have another child while she still enjoyed the flexibility of a school schedule.

In September 2022, she lost the baby in the second trimester and suffered an amniotic fluid embolism during Sebastian's delivery. In the hospital in the middle of the night, Avila went into cardiac arrest after amniotic fluid and fetal debris entered her pulmonary circulation. Her heart did not beat for a full six minutes.

She credits her survival to Sam, who went for help in the middle of the night when she made an unusual sound, and to Dr. Alicia Larsen, her obstetrician and mentor at TCU. Her nurses had also

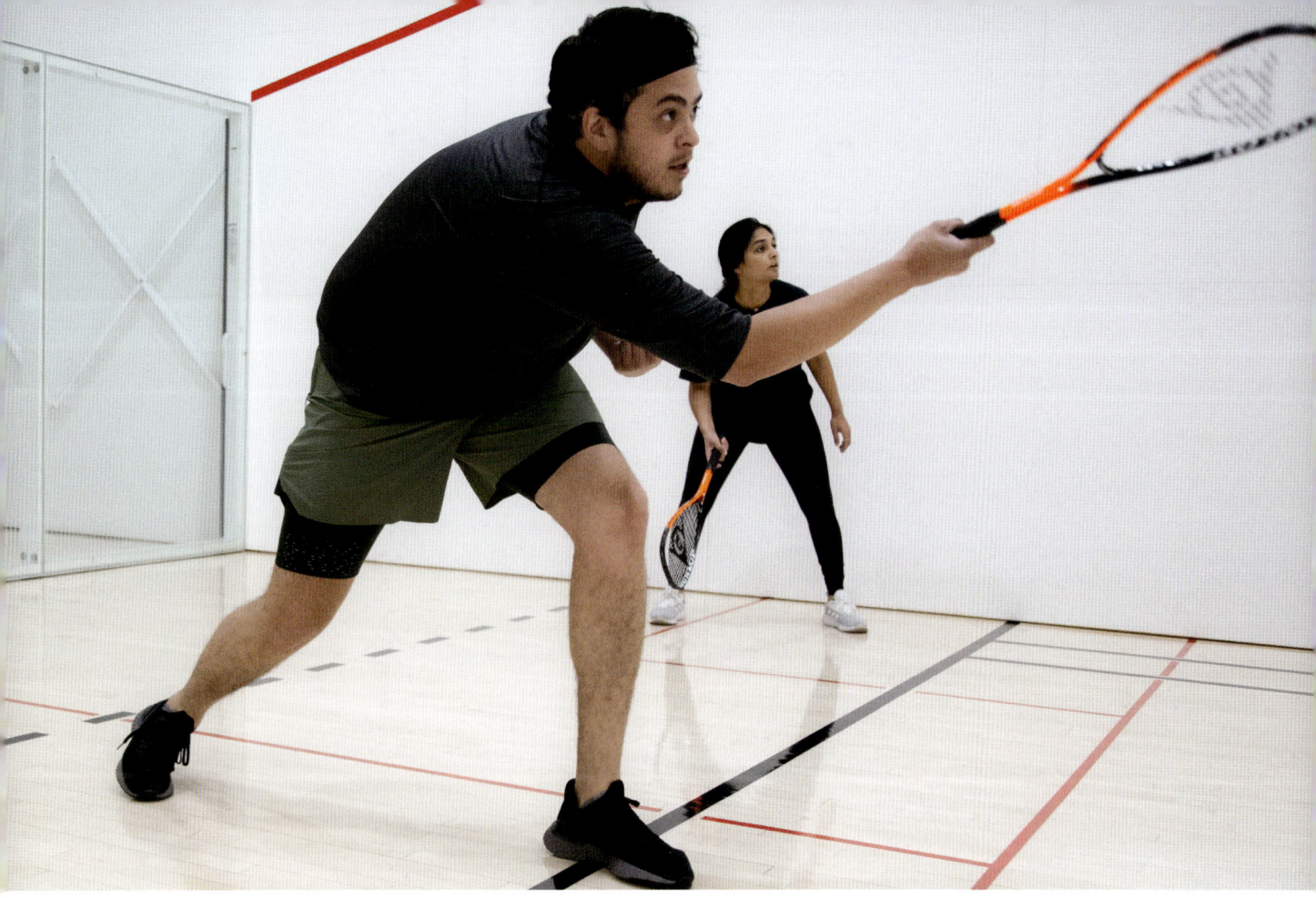

Edmundo Esparza played squash with fellow student Juhi Shah at the TCU Recreation Center. Soon after graduating, he and several classmates attended her wedding in Italy.

practiced a response the previous month to just such a life-threatening situation, another factor she feels was in her favor.

Avila spent a week in the hospital as her body and mind fought to heal. "I don't think there was a single doctor who treated me that had not been my preceptor at some point," she said. "I am 100 percent convinced that if I'd been at a different hospital with a different team, at the very best I would have had some neurological damage."

As she continued to recover, she shortened her scheduled rotation in Temple, Texas, at Baylor Scott & White. Once there, she grappled with grief and fear, which caused significant disruption to her sleep, something she knew OB-GYNs struggle with much of the time. But her confidence during medical school

had grown to the point where she felt certain she could cope with almost anything.

"I am the daughter of hardworking people," Avila said. "I know this is exactly what I'm meant to do with my life."

* * *

The fourth-year medical students began submitting applications in fall 2022 for residency programs. The students believed that beyond test scores and grades, research projects and extracurricular activities could tip the scales in their favor. Depending on the desired specialty, faculty recommended that a student apply to as many as 150 programs.

"Right now, we haven't developed a reputation yet, and we're working very hard on it," said Flynn, who believed the students carried extra pressure as the Burnett School of Medicine's first class.

In deciding which programs to pursue, the students worked with Yolanda Becker, a former transplant surgeon who became the medical school's director of professional career development. Places that prioritize research, such as Brown University and the University of Washington, are classified as academic. Community programs, including Texas Health Harris Hospital in Fort Worth, focus almost entirely on patients.

Kinard set her sights on general surgery at an academic program. In her applications, she highlighted her four years of research in tumor delivery systems designed with nanotechnology. During interviews, she emphasized her student service, which focused on minority representation in the field of surgery. Her work also included a stint as national academic affairs co-chair of the Student National Medical Association, which supports underrepresented U.S. medical students.

Whereas Kinard planned to incorporate research into her medical career, Avila aimed for a top community program. "In my fourth year, I really got to see firsthand that working with women, and hearing their stories, is every bit as rewarding as I'd hoped it would be," she said.

She'd done well on the Step 1 exam in December 2021, which she took while pregnant. Her strong Step 2 results also made her feel confident about earning a spot in a competitive residency program.

During the application process, the bilingual Avila discussed how her MBA would make her a better doctor. She hoped one day to devote 20 percent of her practice to patients on Medicaid or who lacked any insurance. "There's a way to finagle those numbers and keep the lights on," she said, "while still reaching out and giving uninsured or underinsured women access to care."

Shah took geography into consideration when targeting residency programs. His partner, Dr. Shukan Patel, has a successful dental practice in Dallas. The couple became engaged in Europe shortly after Shah graduated from medical school.

Shah's leadership, a selling point to residency programs, was on full display during the annual Out for Health Conference in April 2022. He organized the gathering alongside the medical school's Pride Alliance, which he'd helped found. The conference theme — "If You Only Knew My Story" — dissected the impact of policies and practices relating to LGBTQIA+ patient safety. The conference dovetailed with the medical school's mission to train compassionate doctors.

"The burden is on all of us to make this school great," Shah said.

* * *

Narrative medicine, with an emphasis on writing and empathetic communication, remains fundamental to the Burnett School of Medicine. "It's all about understanding the whole why of the patient, who they are, what they're trying to accomplish, where they're coming from," Kinard said.

The medical school's commitment to patient-centered care shaped how the students thought of themselves within the broader context of health systems.

"Medicine is social work," Losefsky said. "It's not just about disease and treatment. A doctor has to know how patients perceive themselves and the problem, their ability to access care and their ability to make educated decisions.

"When I started at this school, I'll admit I was a little annoyed with the Compassionate Practice®, but I use that stuff all the time," she said. "I've come to a point where I don't think 'Well, it's just a gallbladder,' because this is someone's worst day.

"People listen better when they're being heard,

UCLA T-shirt in hand, Anabel Kruse celebrated her husband's coveted residency placement at the university on Match Day 2023. The couple moved to Los Angeles weeks after graduation so he could start a seven-year program in interventional radiology.

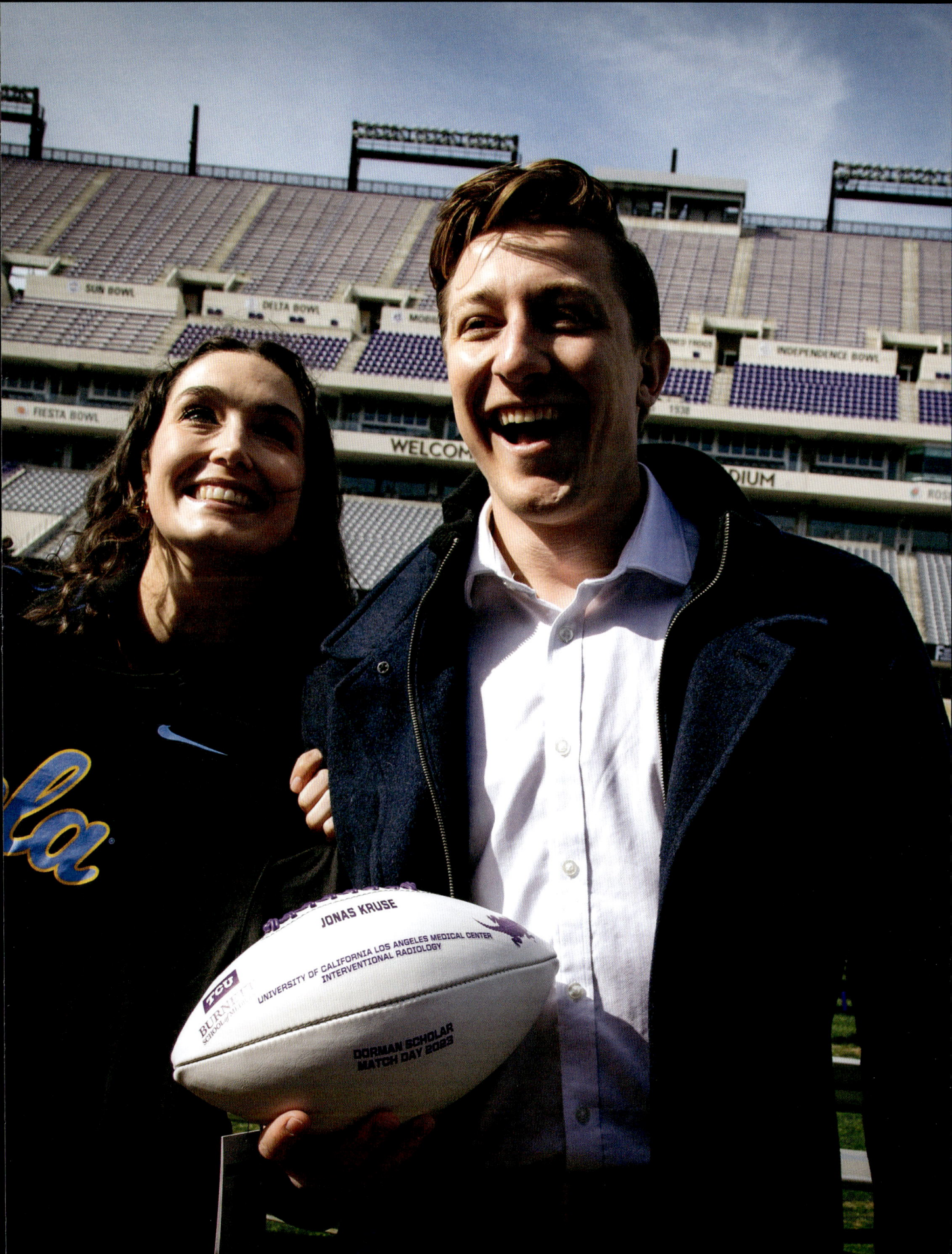

JONAS KRUSE

UNIVERSITY OF CALIFORNIA LOS ANGELES MEDICAL CENTER
INTERVENTIONAL RADIOLOGY

DORMAN SCHOLAR
MATCH DAY 2023

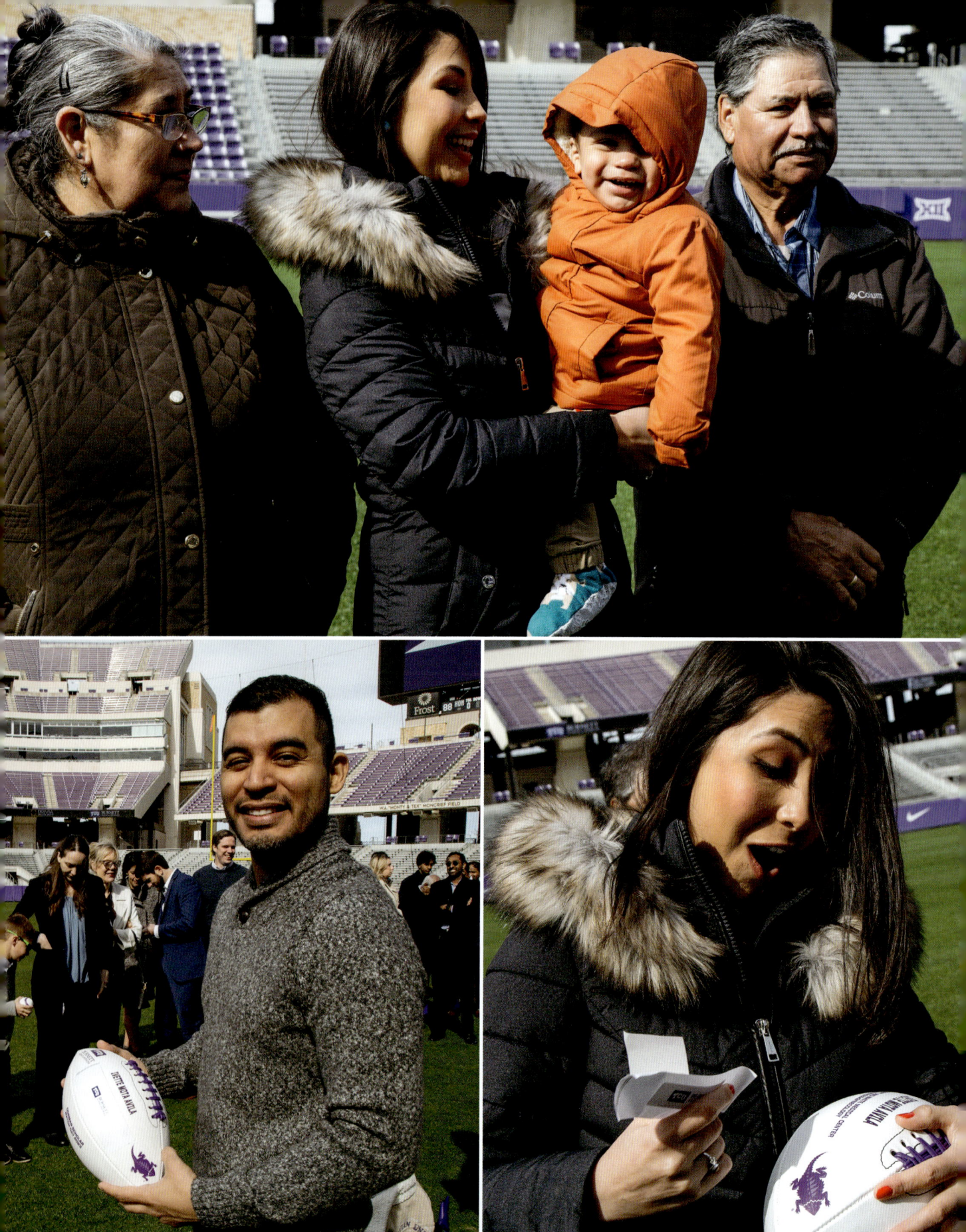

so if you acknowledge that this is a big deal to them while at the same time reassuring them, you eliminate a huge number of problems with miscommunication."

* * *

Residency programs often evaluate thousands of applications to determine which students to interview. Before the pandemic, interviews were conducted in person, meaning most fourth-year students would have to budget for travel. The Class of 2023 instead spent all day, often on Zoom, interviewing remotely for residency spots around the country.

Esparza said he was pleased that he didn't encounter much skepticism or concern about TCU's medical school when he interviewed with prestigious programs at such places as the University of Southern California and the University of Texas Southwestern Medical Center in Dallas.

"I'd get asked about our curriculum with what struck me as a healthy curiosity," he said. "People didn't necessarily know much about us, but they wanted to learn."

"I've been able to sell the new school as a positive," Kruse said. "People are genuinely curious about the type of training we're receiving. The extra time we spend in clinical settings is interesting to them."

Several program directors indicated that Kruse's stellar board scores lent credibility to the quality of his education. Landing in the Top 1 percent for the Step 1 and doing nearly as well on the Step 2 provided an objective way for schools to measure him against his peers.

Losefsky was among those who did interviews in the Harrison Building on TCU's campus or at International Plaza, the medical school's temporary home in southwest Fort Worth until midway through 2024.

"All of the interviews have been so different," she

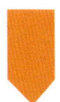

"I've been able to sell the new school as a positive. People are genuinely curious about the type of training we're receiving. The extra time we spend in clinical settings is interesting to them."

Jonas Kruse

said. "Some are very structured, and some feel pretty laid-back."

While interviewers typically asked why the students wanted to pursue a certain specialty and what excited them about a given residency program, the students did field some out-of-the-blue questions.

"The question that shocked me was what was my favorite movie I saw last year," Shah said. "In my head I was thinking, 'Do I go to the movies?' I've been busy!"

Students used the interviews to learn more about a school. They asked about faculty turnover, hospital culture and the city or town where the program is located.

"I only want to go to a program where I feel comfortable asking questions," Avila said. "My top consideration is that I want a place where I can grow and learn."

"I want as much responsibility as a program will give me," Losefsky said.

In February 2023, the students formally ranked the places they'd interviewed with in order of preference; some spent weeks ordering, then reordering, their lists.

Clockwise from top: Avila reveled in the Match Day festivities alongside her parents, Rebeca Mota and Samuel Mota, and her son, Quentin; As the crowd in the Amon G. Carter Stadium cheered, the future OB-GYN ripped off a sticker to reveal she'd matched to her top choice: Texas A&M School of Medicine — Baylor Scott & White Medical Center in Temple, Texas; Sam Avila felt the Horned Frog spirit following his wife's big reveal.

The programs then ranked their pools of applicants. The preference lists from the students and institutions went into the National Resident Matching Program's computerized algorithm.

Across the country, 42,952 applicants matched to 40,375 positions in advance of Match Day 2023. The students learned on Monday, March 13, 2023, whether they had in fact matched, but not where.

Esparza's stomach did a flip that morning when he opened an email congratulating him on securing a slot in a residency program. "This has been such a nerve-racking process going on for so long," he said. "Monday meant I'm going to be a practicing physician."

For many, the buzz of learning that they'd indeed matched lasted less than a day. Then the worry about where they would wind up came back with a vengeance. To distract themselves from the prospect of four more days of waiting, Esparza, Shah and their classmates organized parties, brunches and a field day.

By Thursday, March 16, as family and friends began to arrive in Fort Worth from all over the country, a pervasive sense of anxiety disrupted everyone and everything affiliated with the medical school.

"Thursday was the longest day of my life," Kruse said.

* * *

The Burnett School of Medicine, so dedicated to

Below: Losefsky celebrated her match to a top general surgery program at the University of Louisville with her parents, Pam Bixby and Ron Losefsky. Right: Sunil and Ila Shah, their son and his partner, Dr. Shukan Patel, were all smiles after learning the new psychiatrist would be moving to Denver for his residency program.

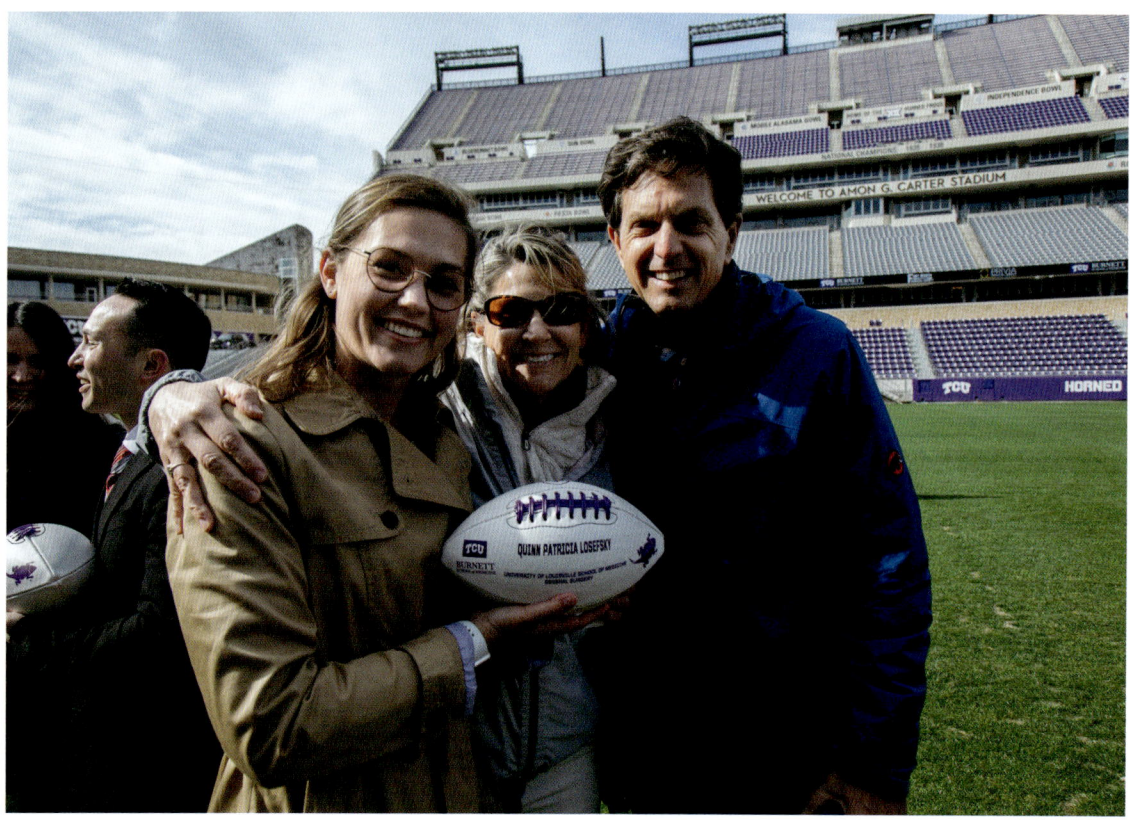

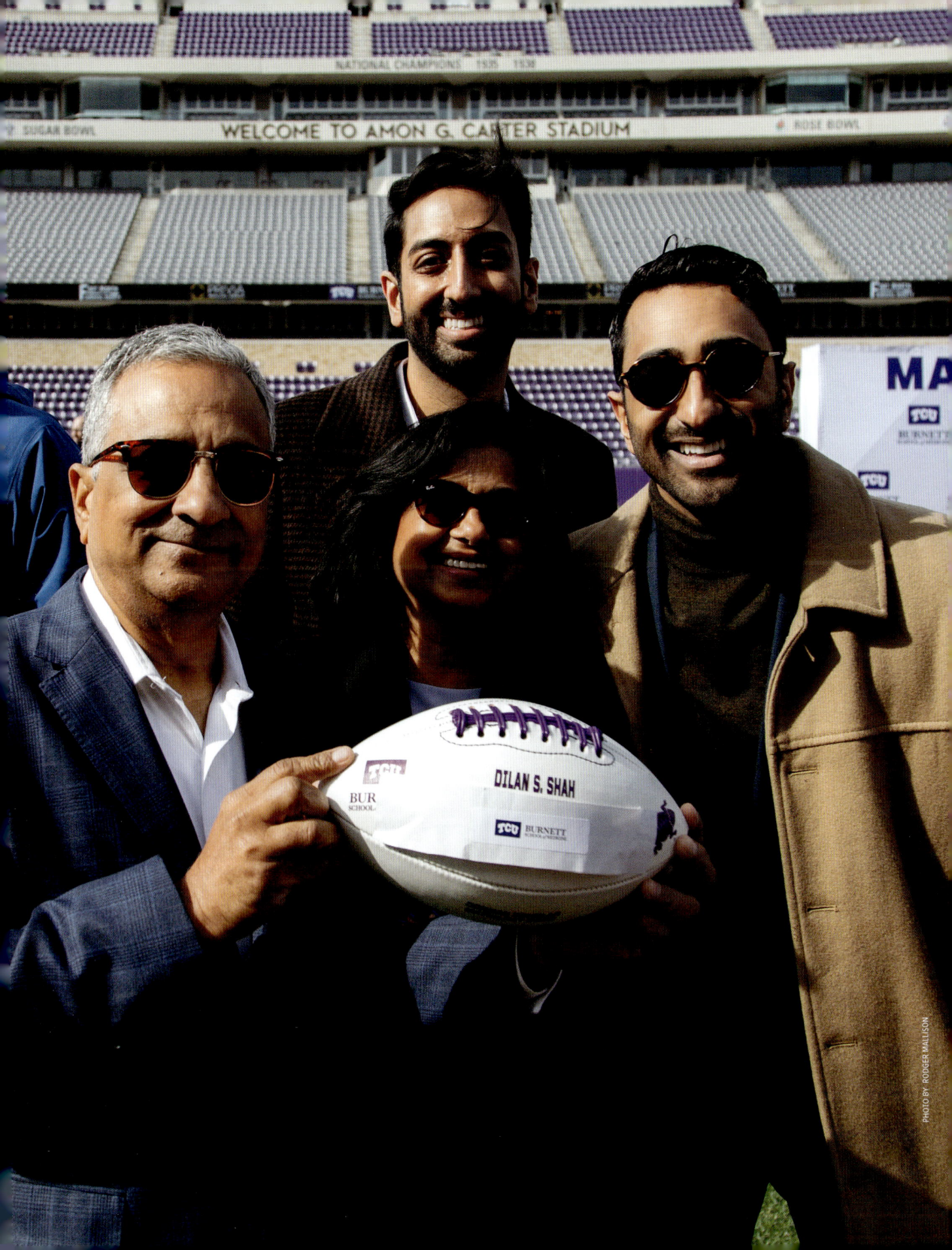

TCU
BURNETT
GENERAL SURGERY
DORMAN SCHOLAR
MATCH DAY 2023
TCU
BURNETT
SCHOOL of MEDICINE

ESPARZA
CALIFORNIA SAN DIEGO MEDICAL CENTER
INTERNAL MEDICINE
AN SCHOLAR
H DAY 2023

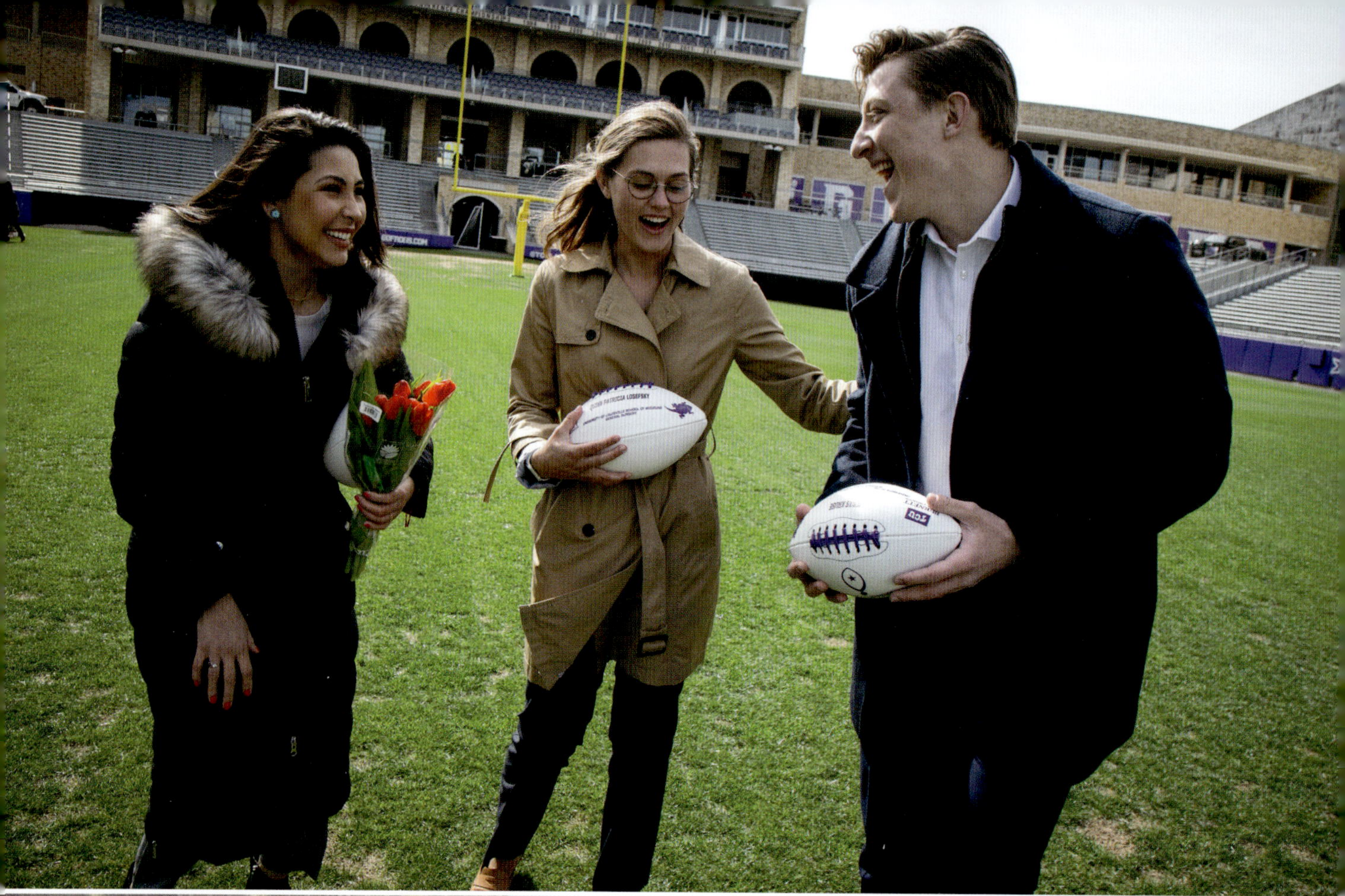

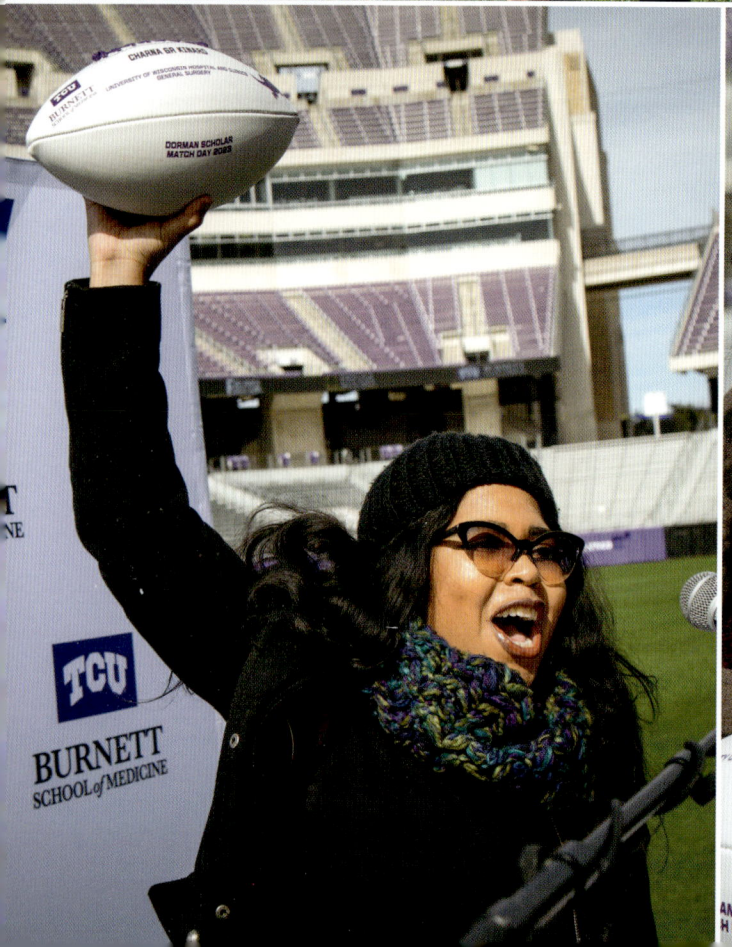

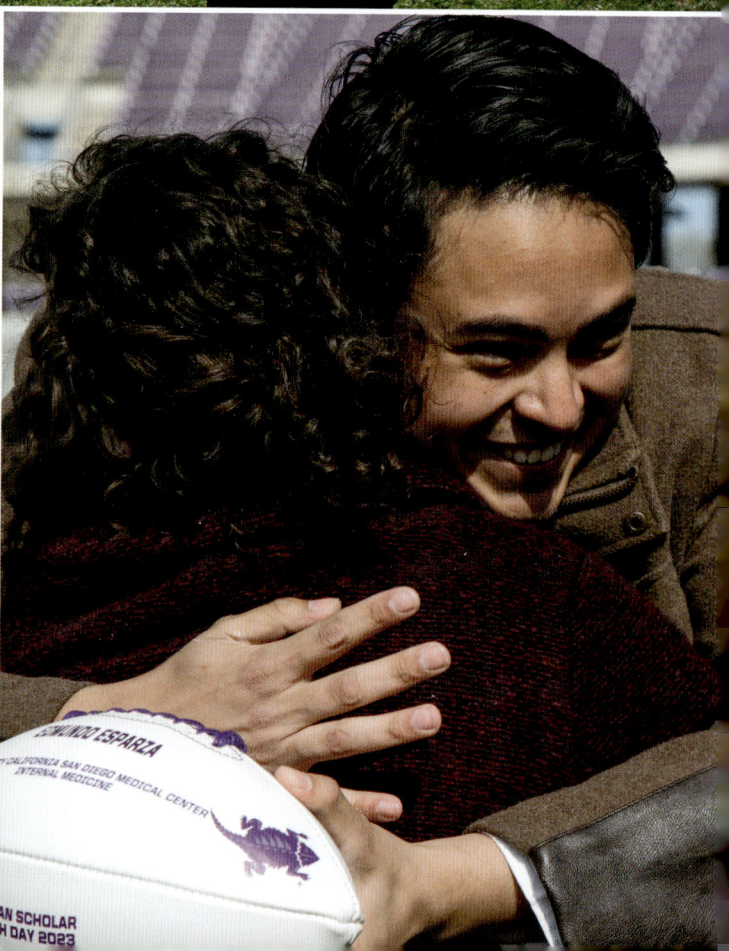

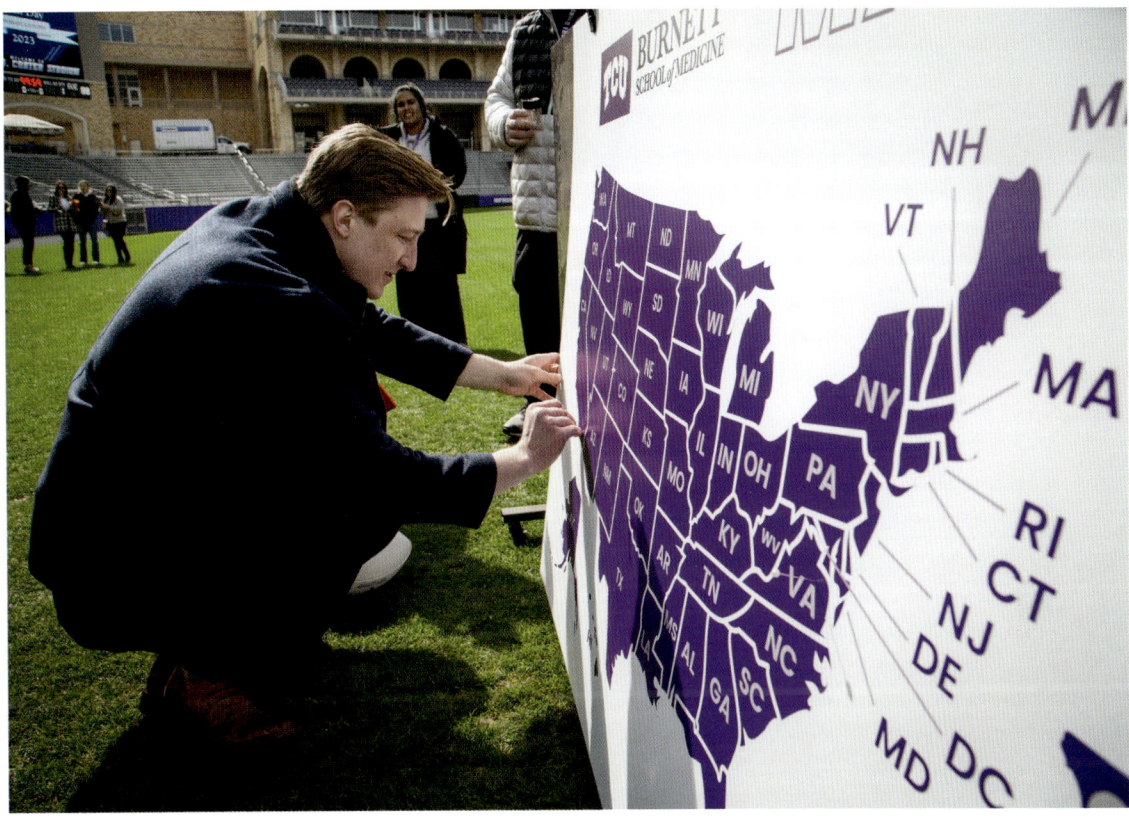

Kruse placed a pin on Los Angeles on the map showing the nationwide residency placements of the Dorman Scholars.

creating a new kind of doctor, took a novel approach to Match Day 2023.

On Friday, March 17, the Class of 2023 processed onto the Amon G. Carter Stadium field with family, friends and physician mentors surrounding them. Many more supporters were in the stands. A cold wind swirled as the 10 o'clock hour ticked away.

As each student stood waiting on the field for the clock to strike 11, a line of people marched onto the grass, each holding a white football. Every football had the name of a student printed in purple ink. Below

the name — and beneath a thick white sticker — was where the student had matched.

The crowd erupted when Natalie Lundsteen, assistant dean of student affairs, announced that 100 percent of TCU's first graduating class of medical students had matched to a program in the United States, a feat for any medical school. A few minutes shy of 11 a.m., everyone in the stadium began counting down. At the cries of one, those holding the footballs tossed them to the students, who ripped off the labels.

Opposite page, clockwise from top: Avila, Losefsky and Kruse celebrated one of the biggest moments of their lives; Esparza couldn't contain his joy at matching in internal medicine at his top choice: the prestigious University of California San Diego Medical Center; Kinard stepped to the podium to announce that she'd matched to the University of Wisconsin, Madison, for her internship in general surgery.

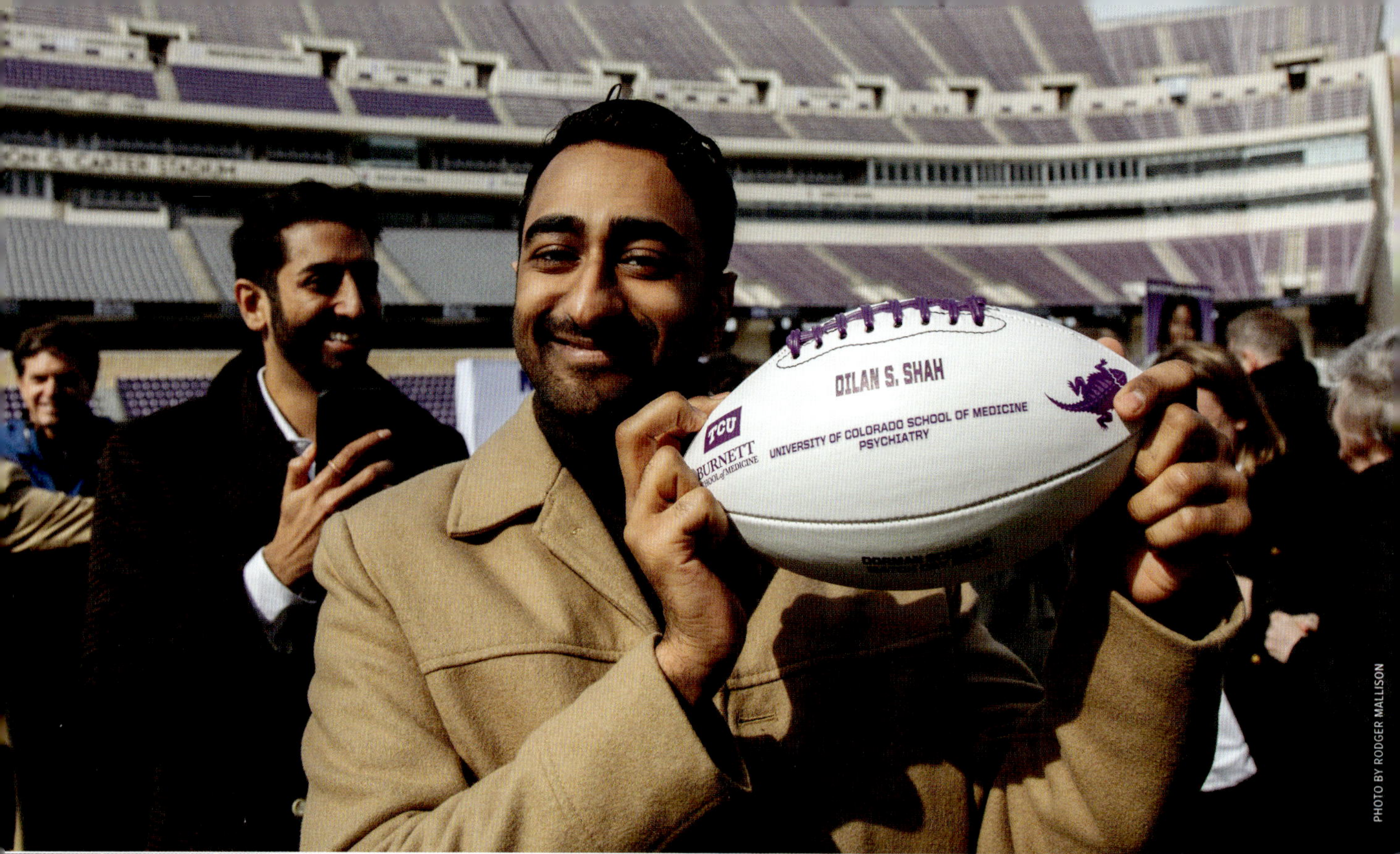

PHOTO BY RODGER MALLISON

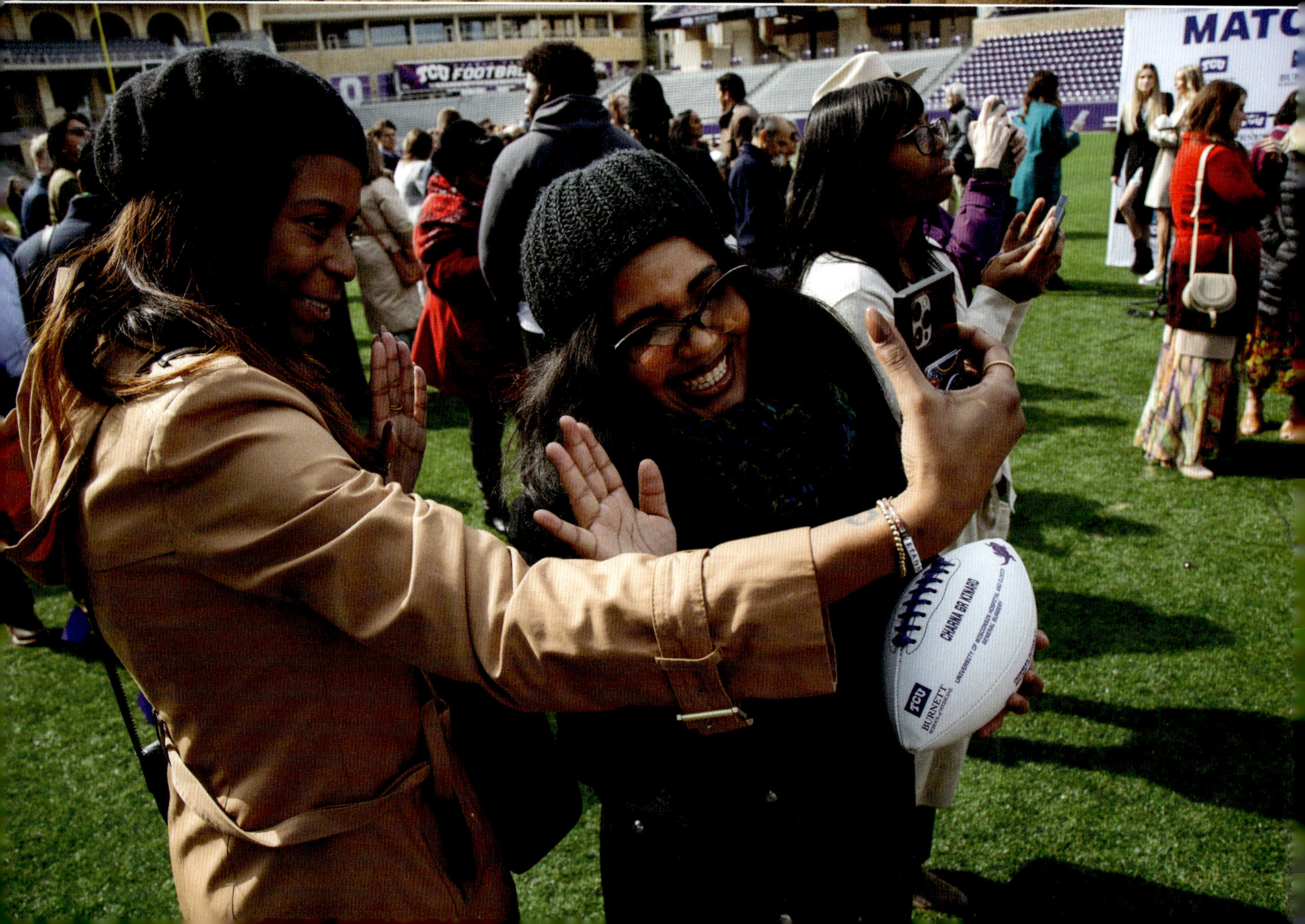

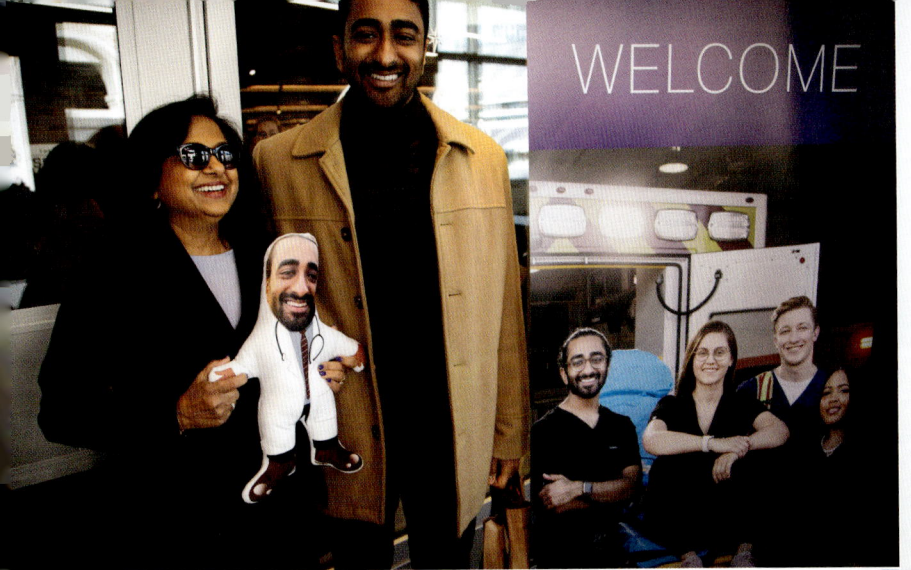

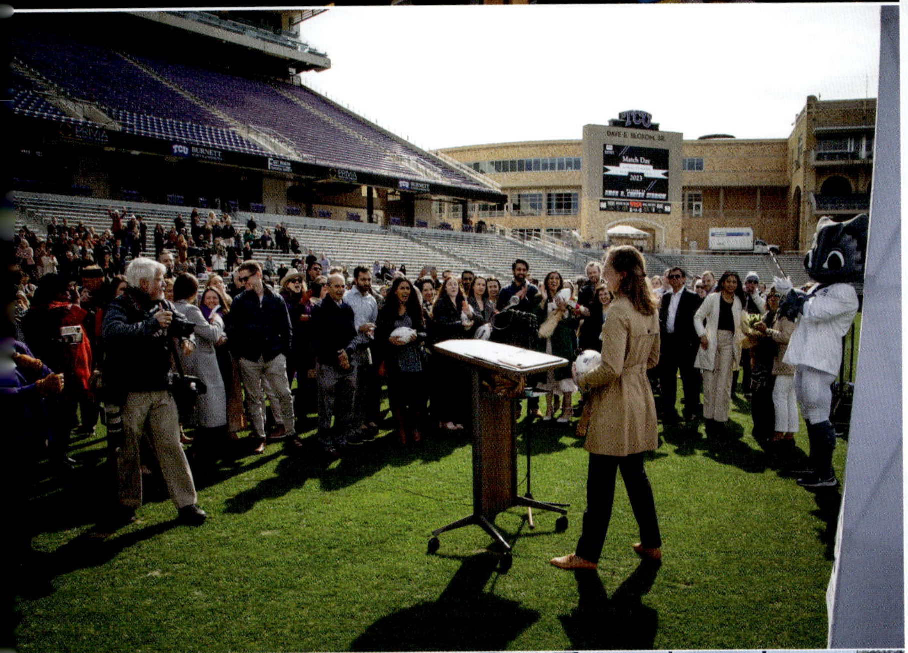

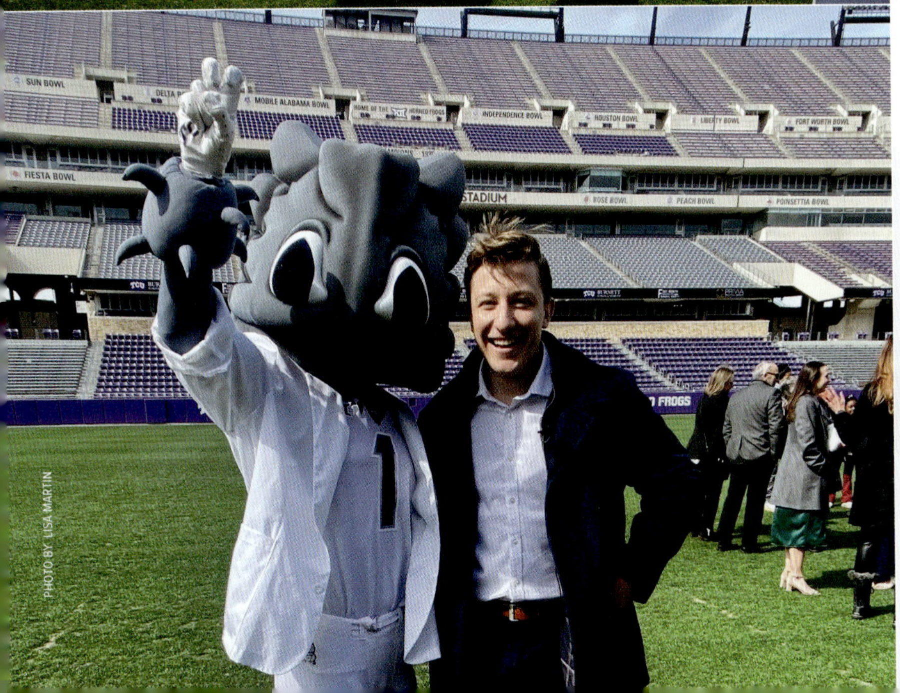

Opposite page, from top:

Shah's football contained his Match Day surprise, a residency placement in psychiatry in Denver.

Kinard took a video call from the grandmother of her longtime best friend, Jasmyne Gorrell.

This page, from top:

Ila Shah held a lookalike doll of her son, Dilan, on Match Day.

Losefsky announced her match at the University of Louisville's rigorous surgery program.

Kruse celebrated his own win, a residency at UCLA, with Super Frog.

PHOTO BY LISA MARTIN

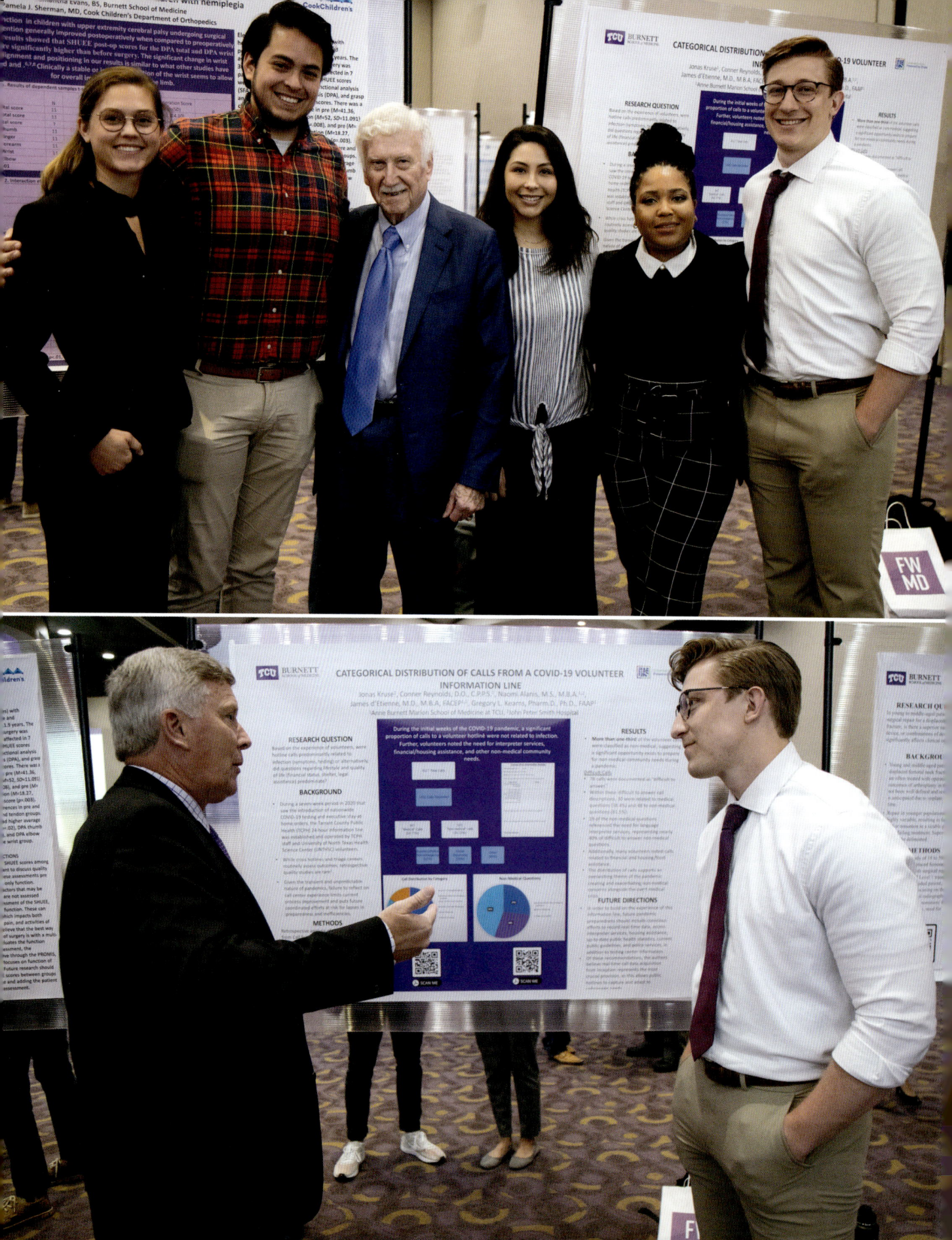

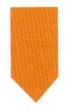

Top: Each student at the Burnett School of Medicine is required to complete a four-year research project. Losefsky, Esparza, Avila, Kinard and Kruse presented their results at the research symposium in April 2023. Attendees included H. Paul Dorman, the Fort Worth businessman and philanthropist who donated more than $3 million to cover the first year of tuition for the Class of 2023.

Bottom: Kruse shared his research with Dr. Stuart D. Flynn, founding dean of the Burnett School of Medicine.

Kruse was a study in delight, breaking into a huge grin. He had nabbed one of three coveted residency spots at UCLA, among the premier interventional radiology programs in the world. It was his top choice.

Other students burst into tears — whether joyful or a release from all the pent-up anxiety — as many began crisscrossing the field to discover where their friends were heading. Most went to the microphone at the podium, where they announced their results to more cheering.

Flanked by her parents with their tear-streaked faces, Avila learned she'd matched to her No. 1 pick at the Texas A&M School of Medicine — Baylor Scott & White Medical Center in Temple. Its maternity center offers the highest level of care in the region. Fourteen-month-old Quentin had thrown his mother the football.

Family members flung themselves at Esparza after they learned he'd matched at the University of California, San Diego. On his away rotation there, he had fallen for the idea of life on the coast and had ranked the coveted program first on his list.

Losefsky, who'd grown up in a saddle, found out she was heading to Kentucky horse country. She was selected as one of nine first-year surgical residents for the incoming class at the University of Louisville, a place with a reputation for intensity. "This is the perfect program for me," she said. "It's a place that's known for rewarding independence. You need to figure out things, which is what I like to do."

Kinard fulfilled her dream of returning to the Midwest by snagging an internship in general surgery at the University of Wisconsin Hospital and Clinics in Madison.

Shah learned he would train for the next four years at the University of Colorado School of Medicine in Denver. "I feel like the universe has been telling me that this is the right answer," Shah said. "I know this is the best place for me."

* * *

The students came together in April for a monthlong transition-to-residency program that addressed everything from professionalism to navigating new hospital systems.

As he prepared to move from North Texas, Shah said he was looking forward to getting to work. "There's such an emotional element to psychiatry as you're parsing through layers," he said, noting the hardest thing about psychiatry "is finding a way to love all patients. Like surgery, it's a skill."

Avila bought a house in Temple and said she couldn't wait to start the next phase of her life. She and her classmates marveled at

> ## "You are now the agents of change. You have the capacity to strive for constant improvements in health, and you have the ability to look to the future for solutions to today's most vexing issues."

Daniel W. Pullin

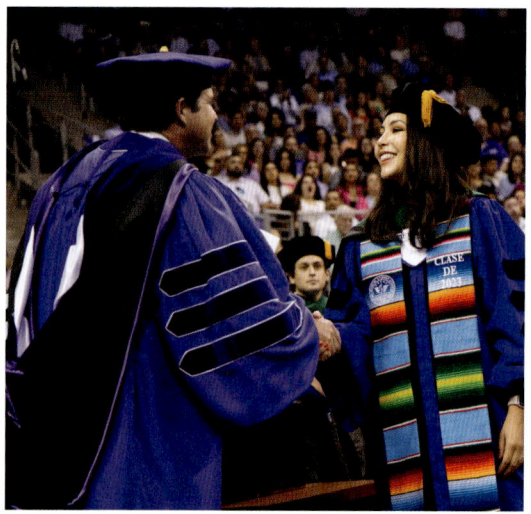

TCU President Daniel W. Pullin congratulated Avila during the hooding ceremony, one day before graduation.

how they'd made it to the end of their four-year journey.

"Med school went by too fast," Esparza said. "I wouldn't go back and relive it because it was too tough, but I made lifelong friends. My advice to my younger self would be never give up, even when you want to."

Esparza's mother and several siblings joined him for the medical school's inaugural hooding ceremony on May 12, 2023.

"You are now the agents of change," TCU President Daniel W. Pullin told the new doctors on stage in the Van Cliburn Concert Hall the afternoon before graduation. "You have the capacity to strive for constant improvements in health, and you have the ability to look to the future for solutions to today's most vexing issues."

Pullin challenged the inaugural graduating class to continue to innovate and work toward improving patient care.

The ceremony concluded with the students taking the Hippocratic Oath, a code of ethics for physicians that dates to 400 B.C. Clad in their purple robes and black velvet tams, the group recited the oath, which includes the iconic phrase "do no harm."

At graduation the next morning inside Schollmaier Arena, the Class of 2023 was honored as the Anne Burnett Marion School of Medicine's first. Each was awarded an oversized MD diploma; the medical school had gifted them with special frames.

Losefsky, who celebrated the milestone with her parents, brother, paternal grandmother, extended family and Gino Piamonte — who became her fiancé in March 2024 — was preparing to leave the university that had been her home since 2015.

"My time at TCU has shaped me into the person that I am and has been some of the best years of my life," she said, "but I do feel like I'm ready to leave the nest."

"I'm floating on air," Avila said. She and Sam were expecting a daughter in fall 2023: Violet Victoria Avila arrived at the hospital where her mom worked, sporting a stunning head of black hair.

After several weeks of post-graduation travel in Europe and South America, Kruse packed up his home in Fort Worth to return to Southern California with his wife and dogs. There they reunited with his parents, stepparents and sister, who had supported him every step of the way.

"The overwhelming feeling is we did it," he said. "The days were incredibly long, and the years zipped by."

Like his classmates, he felt excited for new challenges, people and perspectives.

"I know residency is going to demand more of me, but I'm ready," Kruse said.

"Let's go."

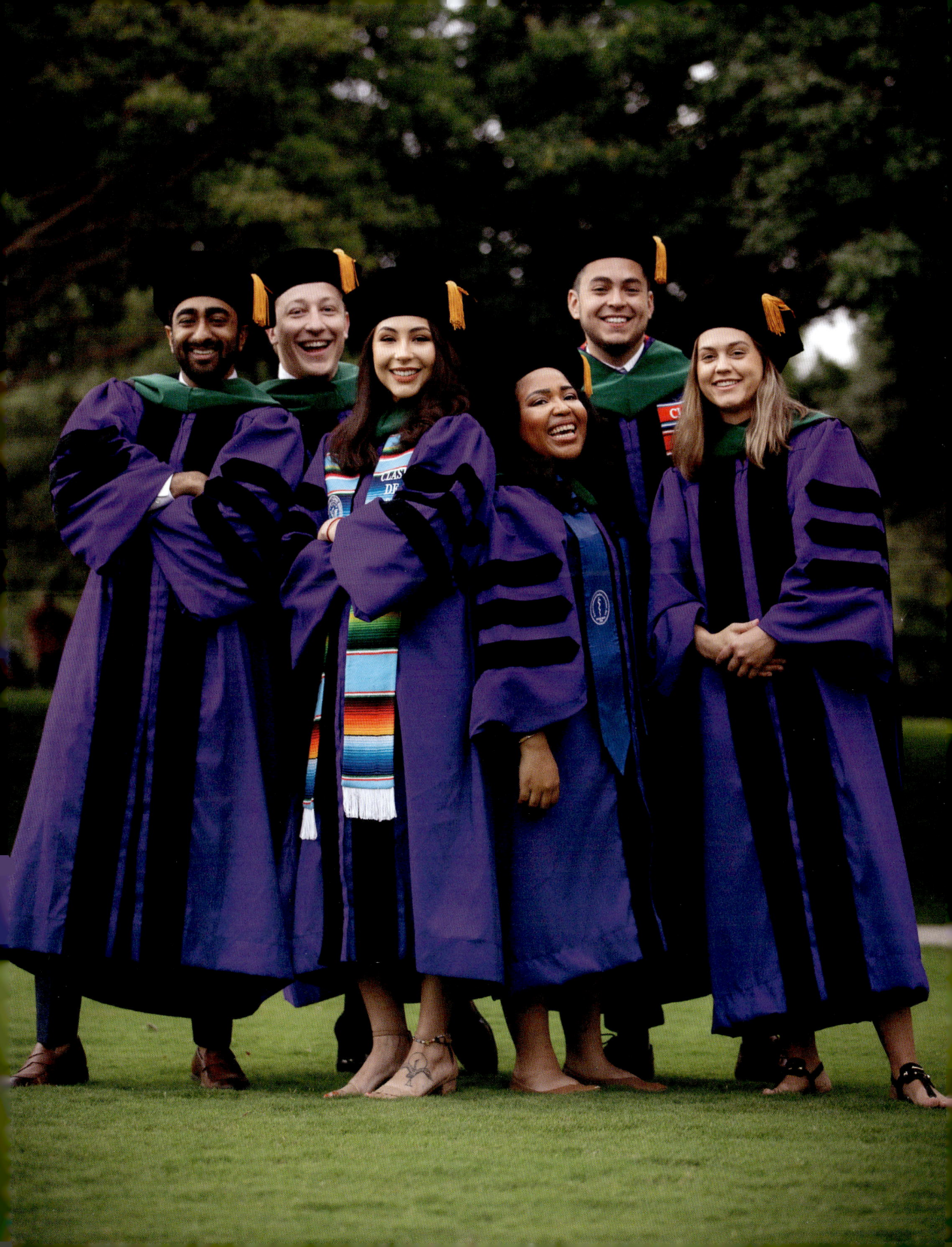

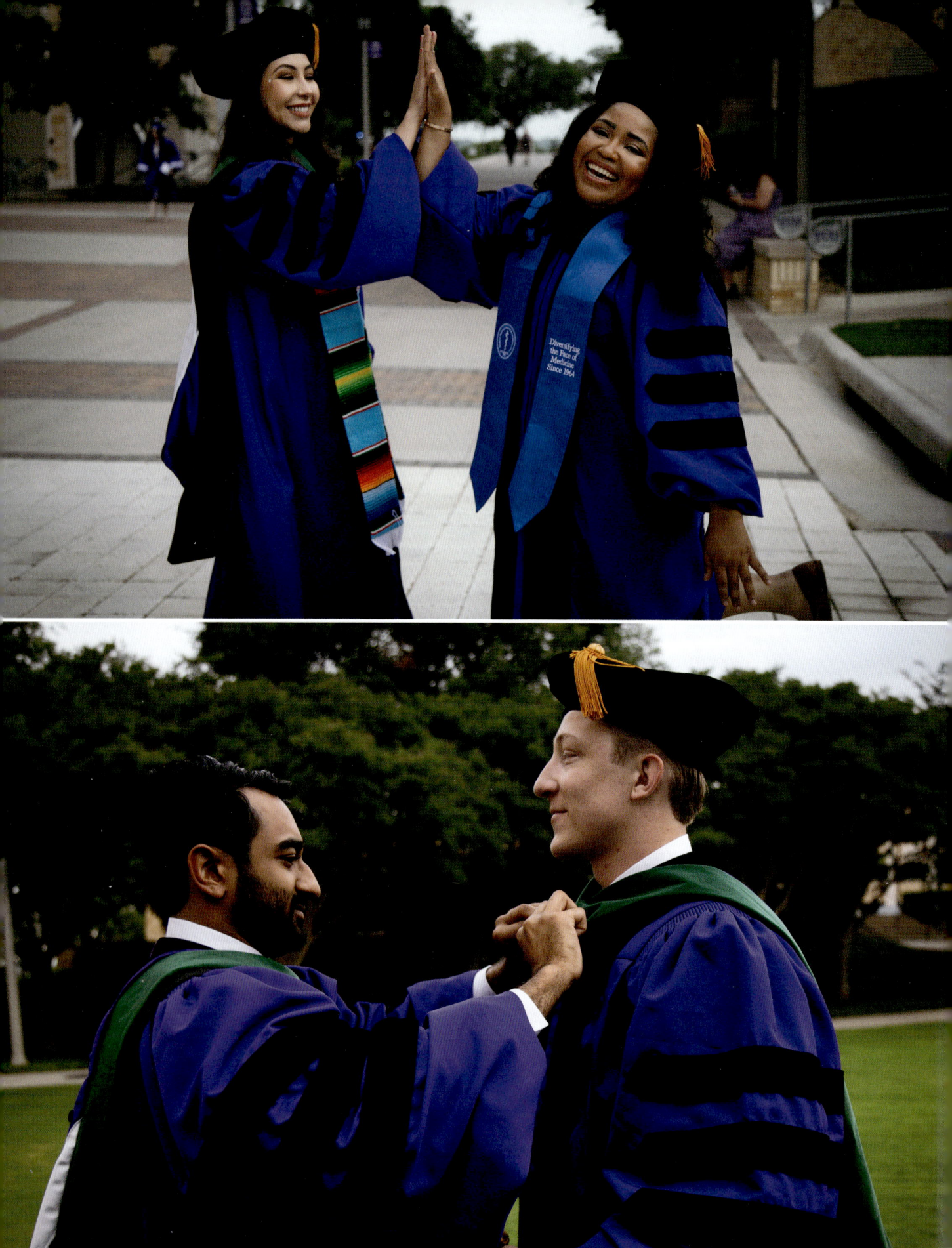

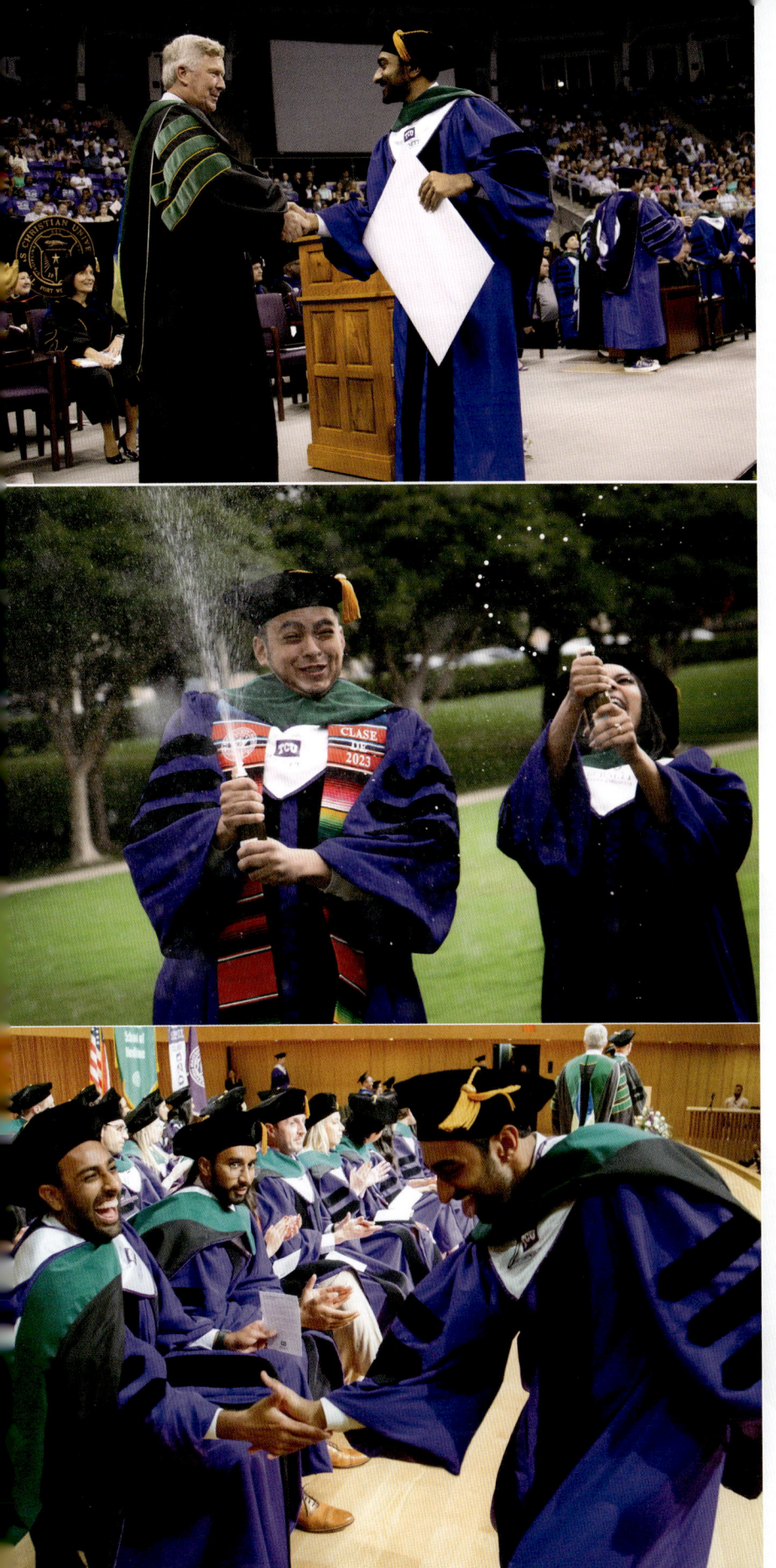

Opposite page, from top:

Avila and Kinard celebrated moments before filing into TCU's Schollmaier Arena on May 13, 2023, when they would be among the first class of graduates from the Anne Burnett Marion School of Medicine.

Shah gave Kruse an assist with the regalia worn by TCU's first 21st-century class of medical graduates.

This page, from top:

Dean Flynn congratulated Shah during the graduation ceremony.

Brand-new doctors Esparza and Juhi Shah uncorked the champagne.

Dilan Shah shook the hand of classmate Sameer Allahabadi at the hooding ceremony. During the event, the 52 graduating physicians recited the Hippocratic Oath.

A Proper Name

Members of the TCU community gathered in the Brown-Lupton University Union ballroom in November 2022 to celebrate the naming of the Anne Burnett Marion School of Medicine.

The Burnett Foundation and Anne Marion made a total of $50 million in gifts to help bring about the vision of a medical school devoted to empathetic communication and technological innovation. Marion's gifts were the largest from a single donor during Lead On: A Campaign for TCU, which succeeded in raising $1 billion by its conclusion in May 2023.

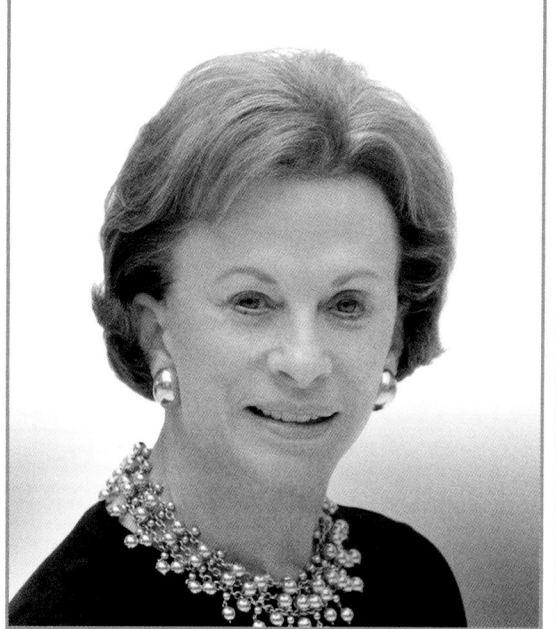

In July 2022, TCU announced the medical school would be renamed the Anne Burnett Marion School of Medicine to honor the late Fort Worth rancher and philanthropist. She was also the school's top benefactor.

COURTESY OF THE GEORGIA O'KEEFFE MUSEUM | © ROBERT WOO

there are still plenty of glass ceilings to break. It is incredibly inspiring to say I come from a school named after such a tenacious, strong-willed woman."

A former TCU Trustee, Marion was the great-granddaughter of legendary cattleman and 6666 Ranch founder Samuel "Burk" Burnett. He was the husband of Mary Couts Burnett, the namesake of TCU's library and the single largest financial supporter in university history.

Marion was an arts patron who founded the Georgia O'Keeffe Museum in Santa Fe,

Special guest H. Paul Dorman was greeted at the naming celebration by medical students Quinn Losefsky, Dilan Shah and Edmundo Esparza. The Fort Worth businessman and philanthropist donated full-tuition scholarships to all 60 medical students in the inaugural class for their first year.

"That gift made an impact," Shah said. "I know my classmates and I will always appreciate what he did for us."

Losefsky kicked off the evening's program by telling the audience that when she graduated in May 2023, she will have earned both her undergraduate degree and medical school degree from TCU.

"I really can't think of a more fitting namesake for our medical school than Anne Burnett Marion," Losefsky said. "As a woman going into the surgical field,

New Mexico. For decades, she supported the Kimbell Art Museum and the Modern Art Museum of Fort Worth.

During her lifetime, Marion also sent "countless young men and women" to college, most of whom were children of ranch employees, TCU Trustee Neils Agather Jr. said. He was the executive director of The Burnett Foundation at the time of her death in February 2020.

"Hers was a quiet philanthropy," he said. "She poured her heart and soul into the ranch and took that same approach with giving."

Toward the end of her life, Marion worked alongside Agather to determine the eventual distribution of her estate. She intended for the ranch, which spans more acreage than Fort Worth, to be sold upon her passing. Taylor Sheridan, the Texan who created the popular TV series *Yellowstone*, led a group of buyers to purchase the Four Sixes in its entirety for an undisclosed sum.

TCU announced in July 2022 that the medical school would become known as the Anne Burnett Marion School of Medicine.

"This generosity empowers us to continue recruiting and nurturing talented and diverse students who are shaping the future of medicine and health care in an abundance of ways," Dean Stuart D. Flynn said.

During the naming festivities, Esparza took to the podium to thank Marion and her family for all they had done for the medical school. He shared a table that night with Mark Johnson, then president of the TCU Board of Trustees, and Johnson's wife, Christina. A $10,000 gift from the couple had supported him during his second year.

Many in the crowd dabbed their eyes as Esparza described his immense gratitude to Marion and to the school.

"You may not understand how much your donations impact us as medical students," he said, "but it does in every way."

From top: Quinn Losefsky addressed the 200 donors and supporters gathered on TCU's campus in November 2022 to celebrate the medical school's new, permanent name; Losefsky and Edmundo Esparza caught up with Dr. Stuart Flynn, the medical school's founding dean, at the naming celebration; Esparza thanked the people who had supported the Burnett School of Medicine and his own medical education.

PHOTOS BY GLEN E. ELLMAN

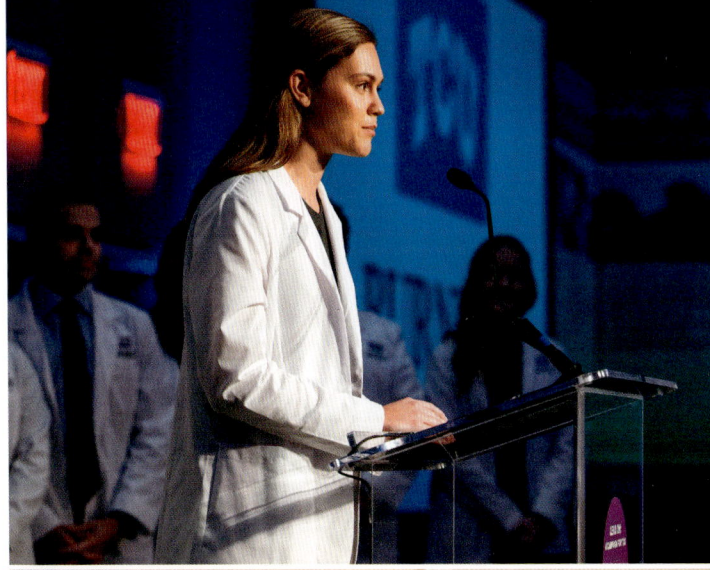

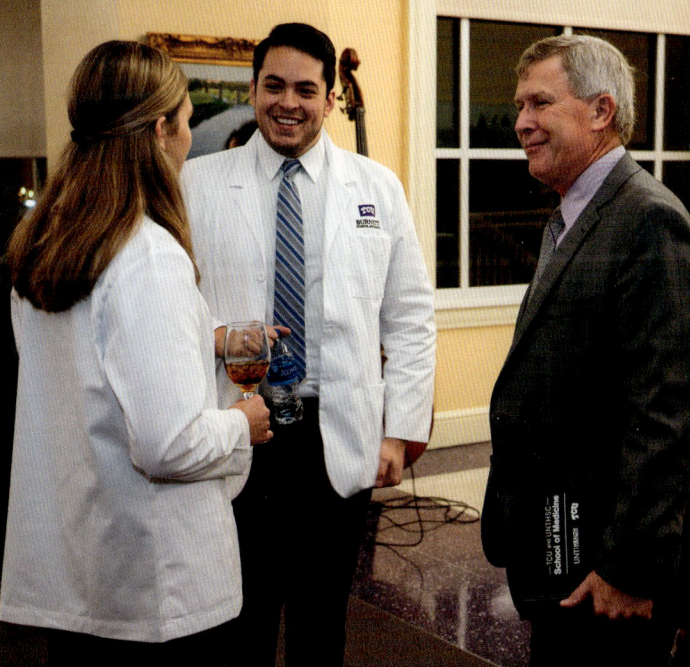

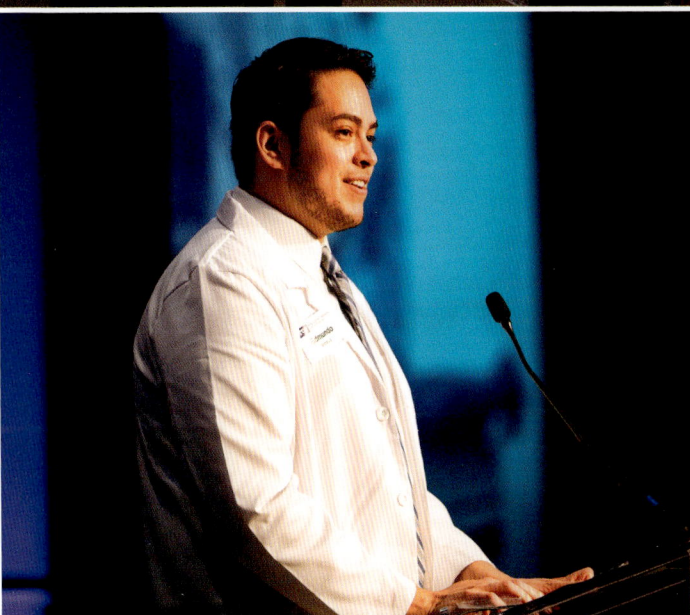

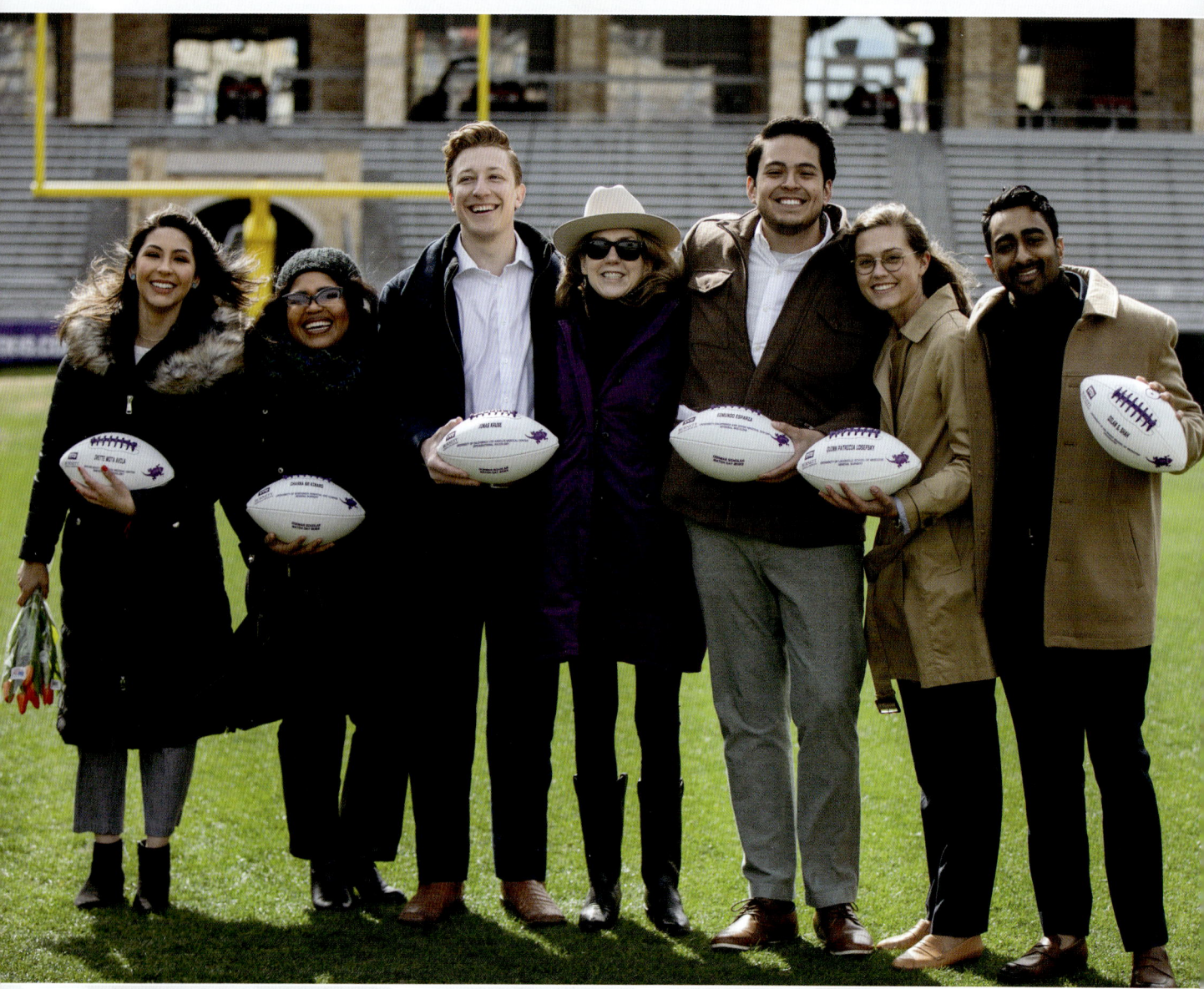

Lisa Martin, center, spent four years chronicling the medical school journeys of Ive Avila, Charna Kinard, Jonas Kruse, Edmundo Esparza, Quinn Losefsky and Dilan Shah. "As a writer, this was a dream experience," she said.

Behind the Scenes

When *TCU Magazine* asked me in 2018 if I'd consider following a group of students through all four years of their education at the brand-new medical school, I didn't hesitate to say yes. My editors could find no other person or publication that had ever done such an ambitious project in terms of duration or scope.

Then came the second thoughts in the months leading up to the day TCU's medical school opened in July 2019. Would the science trip me up? What about the blood? Yet most of my nerves came down to a central anxiety: What if I didn't like one or even most of the students?

Spoiler alert: I like them and did from the start. To a person, they are smart, kind and very good at what they do.

Edmundo Esparza is a 6-foot-4 dimpled gentle giant who answered even the most intrusive questions with patience, humor and grace.

Charna Kinard cares deeply about people and is quick to offer meaningful help.

Dilan Shah asks big questions and doesn't shy away from hard truths, though he's sensitive in how he approaches them.

Jonas Kruse exudes vigor, optimism and a potent intellect, all while rarely complaining.

Ive Avila rallied in the face of tragedy with the kind of personal courage that gives me goose bumps. I'm in awe of her.

Quinn Losefsky, the vivacious baby of our group, dazzled me with her growth mindset. She would take any challenge or setback and extract as much out of it as she could.

During the lockdown months of 2020 and through 2021, I spoke with her more often than anyone outside my immediate family. For the fourth year alone, I took more than 300 pages of notes from conversations with all six.

Though the pandemic prevented me from observing the students with patients as much as I'd hoped or expected, each could recall interactions with such detail and clarity that I felt like I had been there.

I was continually amazed at their passion for service and impressed by their entrepreneurial approach to finding mentors, organizing clubs and activities, and seeking out educational experiences. Like so much in life, medical school is what you make of it.

Their vulnerability could take my breath away. They made me proud.

Over the years, they've gotten to know my story, too. My son, Chip (TCU Class of 2028), and I had dinner with Kruse in New York City in September 2022 while he was doing an away rotation on the Upper East Side. I met Kinard and her mother in Chicago's Loop for dinner that fall.

Early on, when a family member had major surgery, all six students gave me insights and encouragement, calming my nerves.

I have worried about them, cheered their victories and even cried over what life has thrown their way. Through it all, I've felt grateful and humbled at how each let me into their lives. To this day, I swell with pride thinking about who they are and all that they've accomplished at TCU and beyond.

— Lisa Martin

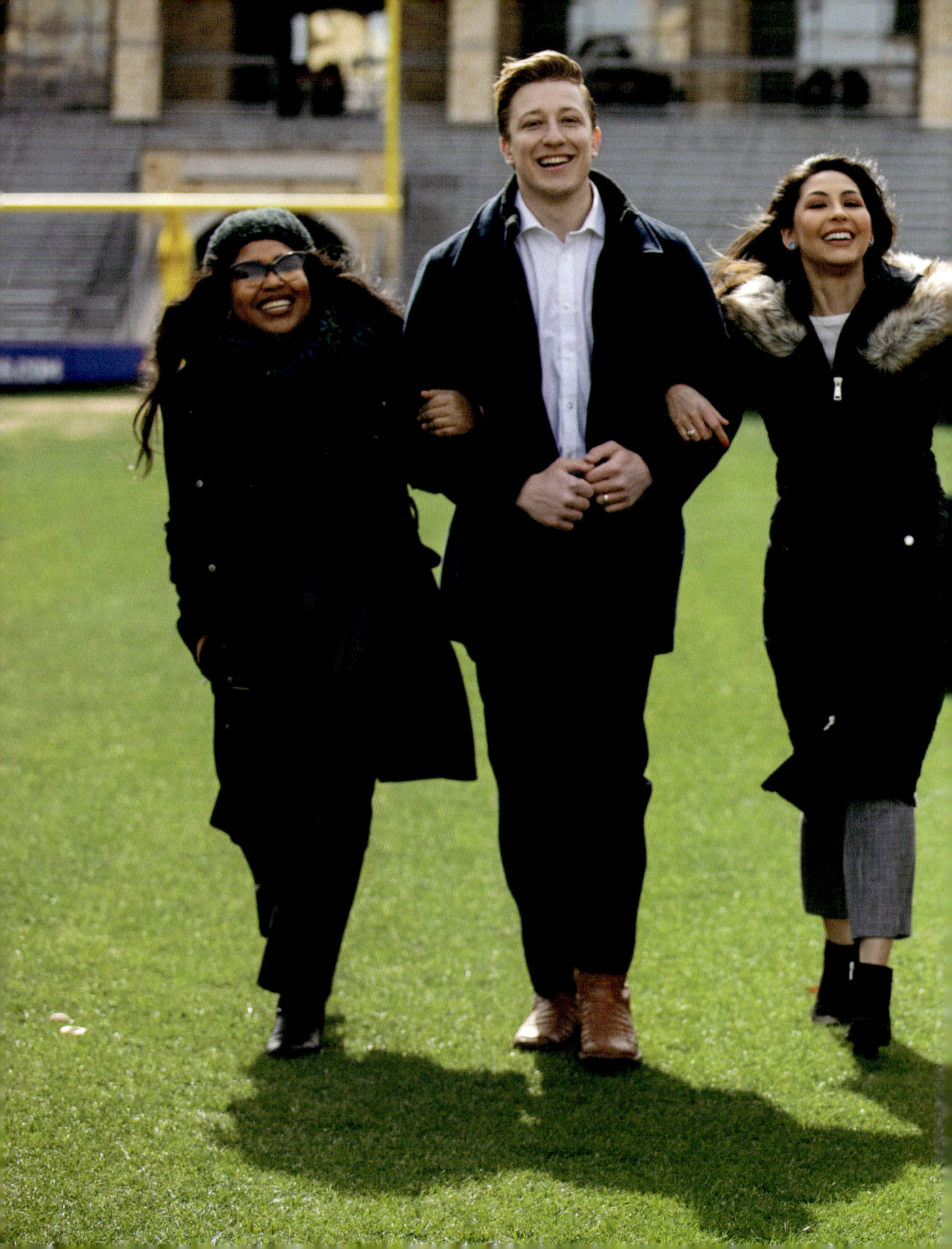

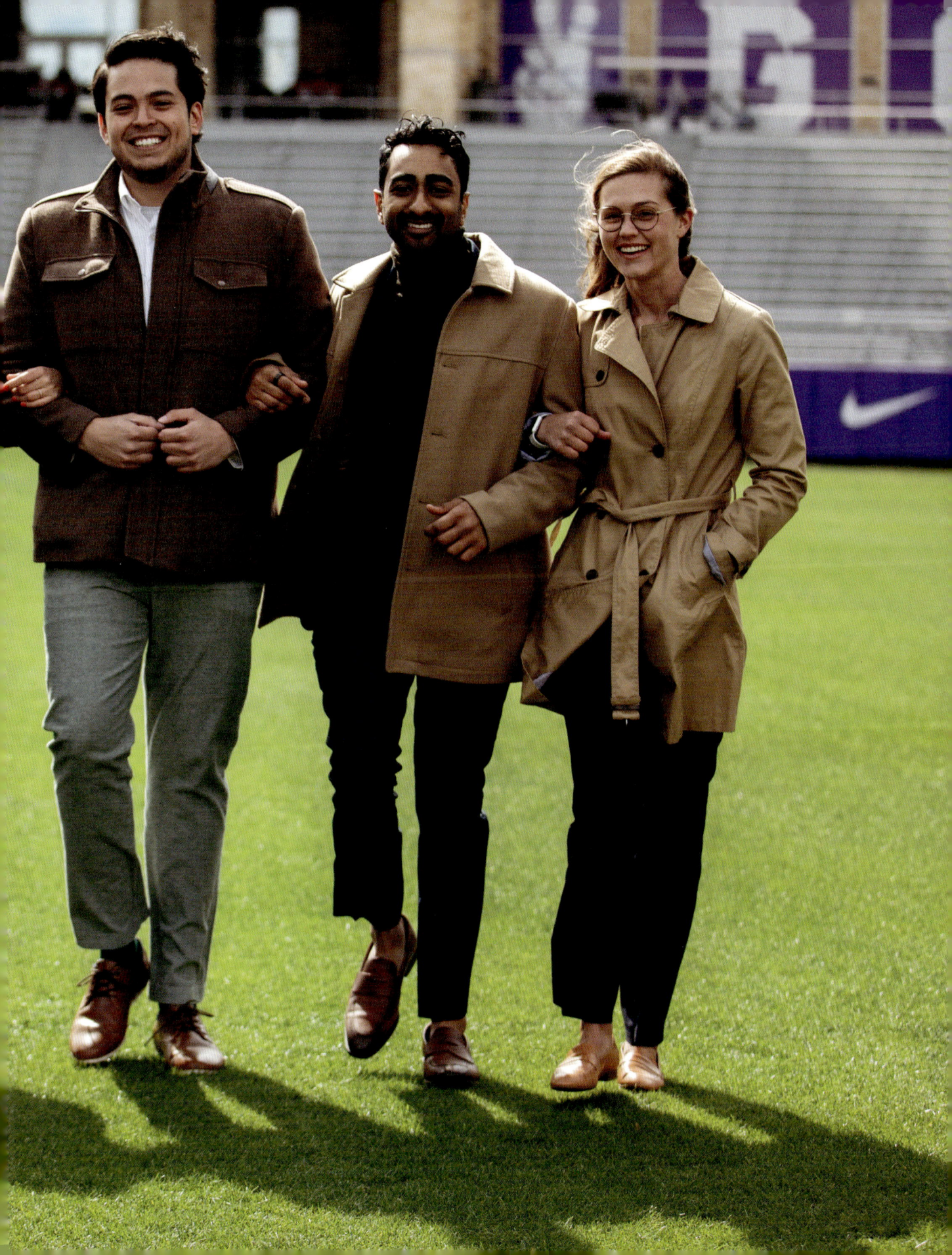

Dedication

To the generous founding donors of the
Anne Burnett Marion School of Medicine at Texas Christian University

Alcon Vision
Amon G. Carter Foundation
Ashley and Greg Arnold
Baylor Scott & White Health
The Bezos Family
Dr. Maureen Murry and Dr. Compton Broders
Mrs. Rebecca and Mr. Jon Brumley
The Burnett Foundation
Cook Children's
Crystelle Waggoner Charitable Trust
Mr. H. Paul Dorman
Mrs. Harriette and Mr. Arnold Gachman
Mrs. Priscilla and Dr. John Geesbrecht
Mrs. Anne Burnett Marion
Martha Sue Parr Trust
Leo Potishman Foundation
The Morris Foundation
Sid W. Richardson Foundation
Thomas M., Helen McKee & John P. Ryan Foundation
Mr. Wade Simpson
Tartaglino Richards Family Foundation
Texas Health Resources
The Walsh Family

Special thanks to anonymous donors

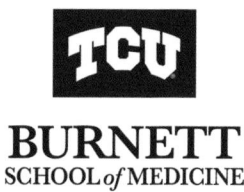

BURNETT
SCHOOL *of* MEDICINE